Weighty Issues

Getting the Skinny on Weight Loss Surgery

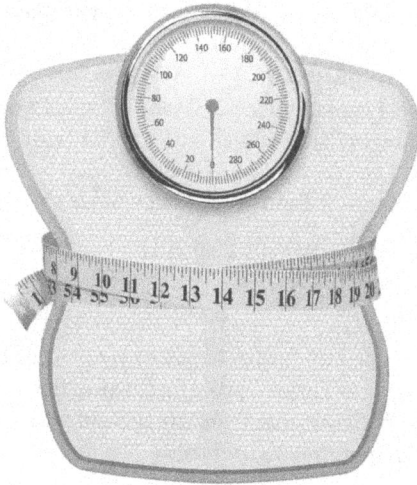

Scott A. Cunneen, MD, FACS, FASMBS

Director of Metabolic and Bariatric Surgery
Cedars-Sinai Medical Center
Los Angeles

and Nancy Sayles Kaneshiro

Smiling Irish Press

WEIGHTY ISSUES *Getting the Skinny on Weight Loss Surgery*
By Scott A. Cunneen, MD, FACS, FASMBS and Nancy Sayles Kaneshiro
Published by Smiling Irish Press,
22647 Ventura Blvd., #219, Woodland Hills, CA 91364
www.weightyissuesbook.com

Publisher's Cataloging-in-Publication data

Cunneen, Scott A.
Weighty issues: getting the skinny on weight loss surgery
Scott A. Cunneen, MD, FACS, FASMBS and Nancy Sayles Kaneshiro
p. cm.
ISBN 978-1-61061-523-5
1. Obesity–Surgery–Popular works. 2. Gastrointestinal system–Surgery–
Popular works. 3. Weight loss–Popular works. 4. Bariatric Surgery Popular
works. 5. Obesity, Morbid–Surgery–Popular works. 6. Gastric bypass–
Popular works. I. Kaneshiro, Nancy Sayles. II. Title.

RD540 .C86 2011

617.5/53 –dc22   2011913473

Book design and cover design by Kirk Thomas, Kirk's Graphics
Printed in the USA

Smiling Irish Press

Acknowledgments

The authors would like to thank a few of the people who helped make this book a reality. Dr. Mona Misra, for her invaluable contribution, constant encouragement and infinite patience; book sherpa (*sherpa?*) Gail Kearns, a genius of organization; and Charlie Hayward, whose horse sense is unerring when it comes to publishing. And many thanks to the patients who bravely came through the doors of Cedars-Sinai to reclaim their health and share their own Weighty Issues with us. Finally, the authors would like to acknowledge each other…they started out as doctor and patient, became writing partners and ended up as friends…not a bad trade.

Table of Contents

Preface

I am a surgeon who specializes in bariatric surgery, that is, I'm the guy who does the gastric bypass and the very popular sleeve gastrectomy operations. OK, I'm a *weight loss* surgeon, but in reality, what I do is better described as *metabolic* surgery. Sure, my patients show up because they want to lose weight, *a lot* of weight, but not just because they think they have a shot at the *Sports Illustrated* swimsuit edition. They come in because of their deteriorating health.

They're diabetic, or hypertensive, at risk for heart attack or stroke, theirkidneys are failing, their hips and knees are shot from carrying so much extra weight. They have gall bladder problems, back problems, sleep apnea. Or any combination of the above. Regardless of age, they do not feel as well as they can or should.

Others come in because they are desperately unhappy. Society is cruel to overweight people. They are stared at, scorned or thought of as weak and self-indulgent. They may not interact with friends easily or have a significant other in their lives. Salaries and employment opportunities are often affected by bosses' attitudes toward overweight workers, thinking them either lazy or a poor insurance risk that will drive rates up.

People who are overweight often feel invisible. They're uncomfortable in their own skin. They're unhappy and unhealthy and all they want is to be heard – and seen – for the person they are inside…and many of them don't even know who that person *is* yet!

Whatever the reason, whatever the physical or psychological malady my patients bring with them, the common thread is that they want to "fix it." *Now*. They've tried *everything*, they tell me, and now they need help.

I don't offer the quick fix. Weight loss (or metabolic) surgery *isn't* the quick fix. In fact, it requires a lot of hard work and a lifetime commitment. However, a majority of gastric bypass and sleeve gastrectomy patients are able to significantly improve their health in a very short period of time. Diabetic numbers go down almost immediately for these people, many of whom have their medications drastically reduced or even eliminated following surgery. Also reduced for these patients is the increased risk of heart attack, stroke and kidney failure associated with out-of-control diabetes. That can translate into *years* of increased life expectancy.

Losing weight lightens the load on the joints as well, helping patients to get moving, to exercise, perhaps for the first time in their lives. And, of course, exercise promotes cardiac health and increases lean muscle mass which, in turn, helps burn calories more efficiently. So that's what we call a win-win*!*

Probably the most important thing to do when considering weight loss surgery is to find a program that supports *you*. For example, our program at Cedars-Sinai Medical Center in Los Angeles puts the emphasis on patient education and evaluation. Once a person completes an initial consultation with a surgeon and meets the physical criteria for surgical candidates, that's when the real work begins. Our patients go through an extensive course of on-site education plus psycho-social evaluations with professionals who determine if they have the mindset for success, in addition to extensive lab work and tests to evaluate heart, lungs and anything that would make them high-risk for surgery. This process can take three to six months. Then, following surgery, we offer support groups that help patients adapt to their new lifestyle and stay on track for the long term. People who go through our program know they aren't going through this experience alone. They've got doctors, nurse practitioners, psychologists and dieticians standing by for them, in addition to the many friendships that are forged at our support groups.

Please don't think that if you are investigating surgery, that somehow reflects negatively on you. I hear so often that patients feel like failures because they haven't been able to get a handle on their weight on their own. There's often guilt because diet and exercise haven't worked for them. Of course, surgery should not be taken lightly. Even though these operations have become more and more safe in recent years, it's still surgery and there are risks associated with it. What you need to determine, with the help of your primary physician, is if the risk of being severely overweight is greater than the risk of surgery, and if you are willing to make the necessary commitment for long-term success.

It is my hope that this book will tell you what you won't find in the vast sea of online information where much of what you read isn't vetted for accuracy and should be taken with a grain of salt. Here, I have compiled the most often-asked and important questions my patients pose while they are in the decision-making process, getting ready for surgery or recovering from it. These are issues I address with my patients in the exam room or in my office, where they feel comfortable speaking freely. They are the subjects that come up over and over again in the pre-surgery and post-surgery support groups we offer. These are the questions I face at "Ask the Doctor" sessions, as well as the topics our post-surgical patients cover when they "pay it forward" to those whose surgery is in the future.

This is not an *everything you ever wanted to know about weight loss surgery* book. It's an *I wish my surgeon had the time to answer more of my questions* book. I hope you will use these discussions as springboards for chats with your own doctor. Ask the questions – all of them – the tough ones, the icky ones, the personal ones.

Losing weight to reclaim your health requires a huge commitment and a complete change of lifestyle with regard to food. Is this the easy way out? Nope. It's a long, arduous process, requiring a lot of hard work and dedication.

In the long run, is it worth it? You bet it is!

Dr. Scott Cunneen

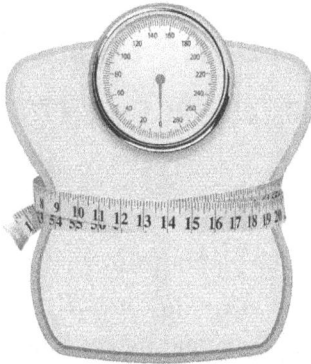

Generally Speaking…

They say that knowledge is power, and no truer words were ever spoken, especially when people are in the process of making life-changing decisions. My patients come in with a wide variety of experience and a whole panoply of questions, most of which boil down to "how do I know if surgery is for me and do you think I can really do this?" We know that the hardest step is that first one through our door and we want to make sure they get the answers they need. Here are some of the general questions we hear most often.

What are the basic types of weight loss surgeries?

A wide spectrum of surgeries exists in the weight loss arena today, running the gamut from what they call *restrictive* operations to those that are *malabsorptive*. The restrictive surgery takes your stomach and makes it smaller, so that food moves more slowly through your stomach. Everything is processed normally after it goes through your stomach in a restrictive operation since we don't rearrange the intestines.

On the other extreme, in the malabsorptive category, your mouth is hooked up to your colon…food goes virtually from your mouth straight into the toilet, bypassing almost the full length of the intestines so you that can't absorb most of the nutrients or the calories in the food. Most surgeons don't do those operations anymore because they're too extreme and the risk is too great for the benefit for most patients.

The good news is that today, somewhere in the middle are the operations like the **sleeve gastrectomy (or gastric sleeve)** and the **Roux-en-Y gastric bypass** (named for a 19th century pioneer in surgery and the configuration the surgery accomplishes), both combining a significant dose of hormonal manipulation with the restriction to get the desired results. This means we've made your stomach smaller, so you have to eat differently, slow down and chew your food well. At the same time, your *head* is less hungry so you can comfortably eat less. These are the operations that have proven to have the best risk-benefit ratio.

With bypass, the small intestine is cut about 1½ to 2 feet below the stomach and is attached to the new, small stomach pouch we've created. The other part of the intestine is reattached so that the bile and other digestive juices can flow easily and mix with the eaten food. Food moves from the new stomach pouch directly to the lower part of your small intestine, bypassing the old stomach and first part of the small intestine. While bypass definitely offers more guaranteed weight loss than most procedures, because we're cutting and rearranging things, there's a little more risk with that procedure, and taking vitamins becomes non-negotiable after surgery and for the rest of your life.

Whereas early restrictive surgeries relied on fixed-sized rings to accomplish their goal, in later years the restriction became *adjustable* with the use of the gastric band. It became evident, however, that one risk of banding is the possibility of not losing all the weight you want because you can cheat it easier (thereby leaving the band a distant third in popularity of weight loss procedures). If you choose to drink primarily high-calorie liquids, for example, I can never make a band tight enough to stop the liquid since I have to leave enough room for you to drink water and stay hydrated. With bypass, eating certain types of food will make you sick and you're sort of forced into weight loss by default, and the sleeve limits your intake by reducing the size of the stomach to a fraction of its original capacity. For those whose weight loss goals are more modest, banding may still be appropriate, since it allows for less manipulation with the surgery and is less invasive, and can help you to get to your goal, enabling you to get the weight off so that your diabetes is better controlled, your hypertension, your sleep apnea -- all those things we call *co-morbidities* or illnesses that are related to your being overweight -- all those things reverse, and you don't have to have the maximum amount of weight loss in order to accomplish that. You can lose 40% or 50% of your excess body weight and get those health benefits.

The more recent choice we mentioned added to the mix – one with achievable weight loss slightly less than bypass, but enough to pretty much replace the band, is the **sleeve gastrectomy**, which is basically the removal of about 90 percent of your stomach, meaning you wind up with a long tube that connects the esophagus to your small intestine that is about the same diameter as the esophagus. What you lose is the reservoir function of the stomach. The size of your new stomach is about 60cc, or about the size of a banana or a quarter of a can of Coke, so it fills up fast. Also, it has become clear that our intestines are not just hollow tubes that absorb things and carry things in transit; there are hormones that are released in the intestines that affect hunger and how we process foods and sugars, so hunger is regulated by more than just the amount of food we eat. Different kinds of food trigger those hormones, and what remains of the stomach after surgery affects hormone levels which allow you to eat less, with a little bit less manipulation of the intestines than gastric bypass. The sleeve gastrectomy is being widely used and has become a staple (pardon the pun) in the bariatric arena.

The risk factors of a sleeve are about the same as with a bypass. When you cut away the majority of the stomach you have a big, long staple line in the stomach, and if that doesn't heal well, leaks can occur and that's when you have the potential for infection. And, if you happen to have diabetes, you might not heal as quickly as you should. So, while people do like the certainty of the weight loss, if you're diabetic, if you're older, if you're severely overweight, all those things contribute to the risk.

In short, most of the weight loss operations today combine a little bit of restriction and hormonal manipulation in order to get you there, rather than go to one extreme or the other.

All of these surgeries are currently done **laparoscopically**, that is, using instruments through very small incisions rather than the necessity of stem-to-stern incisions associated with abdominal surgery years ago. Recovery time has been shortened and risk has been significantly reduced with the use of these minimally-invasive procedures.

If you search the Internet, you may find several more options that people are accessing to help with weight loss. Many are still investigational and most achieve less weight loss than the procedures we just reviewed.

Aren't people who opt for weight loss surgery just looking for the easy way out?

You know, most people who come into my office for weight loss surgery have been overweight their entire lives. They've been on every diet known to man. The conventional wisdom in society is that people who are overweight are just self-abusive. It's generally thought that they just don't care about themselves, that they just don't have enough character to suck it up and go on a diet and lose the weight. After decades of following people to see how they did on diets, however, the consensus now is that diets don't work for more than six months to a year. And at the end of the year, the net loss is often minimal.

In our environment, people *collect* calories, and the majority of us collect more calories than we give up. We call it an *obesogenic* environment…and now it's often referred to as a *diabesigenic* environment because diabetes and obesity are going hand in hand. So, no…it's not the easy way out, it's often the *only* way out for people who qualify for surgery. And if you continue to tell them that a regimen of diet and exercise is the only way to go, then all they're going to do is develop all the obesity-related health problems and never really get the weight off.

We know that the key to success for our patients is the operation *plus* the diet and exercise, so believe me, there is no easy way out. Ask anyone who's had weight loss surgery. They'll tell you they thought it would be easier than it is, but they're doing a lot of work to lose the weight and maintain the weight loss.

Is *there a pattern that you hear from your patients day in and day out as to why they're considering surgery?*

Nearly everyone I see tells me they've generally had a weight problem their entire lives. They've tried everything and nothing has given them lasting success. Somehow they've been exposed to the idea of surgery. Some know a little about it, some know a great deal, but for the most part, they all want their lives to be improved. Women, in general, are more proactive in terms of improving or maintaining good health.

We often see men after they've developed more problems, when their primary physicians have told them there are health-related problems that need to be addressed. They're at risk for developing diabetes. They're starting to have blood pressure problems. They're forced to take medication now, and some of these medications may have some side effects they may not like. And a lot of these guys, because obesity runs in families, may have seen what happened to their fathers or grandfathers and they see themselves going down that same path. And they didn't see a happy ending. So they come in trying to stop it. They know that all the conventional things like dieting haven't worked out, and they're coming in for what they see as the next step up.

Or the *only* step up.

Do you think people need to give it a good try on their own before they have surgery?

Most people will come in and say they've tried and failed and tried and failed and tried and failed. There is a group of people out there, however, for whom concern for their weight has never really been an issue – more men than women, I would think – who wake up at fifty and find they're diabetic, they're hypertensive, and now their doctors are telling them they have to lose weight. For a lot of men it might also be the issue of mobility, meaning their knees are gone, along with diabetes and high blood pressure, and many of their friends are going through the same thing. All of a sudden it's not as cool to be overweight and it's really hampering their lifestyle. These people may never have dealt with a serious weight loss effort before and all of a sudden, the number of pounds they need to lose is daunting.

The majority of people, however, will tell you they've tried dieting at least once before they talk to a surgeon. I think that what's clear in the literature is that once you achieve the weight that allows you to qualify for surgery, diet alone is not going to keep it off. People who find themselves at that weight have bodies that are just wired a little bit differently. Anyone can put on twenty or thirty pounds almost without looking, but it's unusual for people who can succeed with a diet to suddenly find themselves a hundred pounds overweight – or more. In other words, those who can take care of it sooner, usually do.

It seems like the obesity epidemic is worse in this country than anywhere else, doesn't it?

Well, it was. In Third World nations, we have people starving. But what is happening as the western diet is adopted and traditional menus are discarded throughout various parts of the world, obesity follows. In this country, we don't have that problem, we have the opposite problem. Our society as a whole spends *less* on food proportionately than ever before, and it's mostly calorie-dense food now – a lot of calories in a small package – so it's a problem. Even with all the health information available to us, we're heavier than we ever were, with diabetes and other weight-related diseases at epidemic levels.

Obesity has actually become our form of malnutrition.

Do most people show up with a minimum of 100 pounds to lose?

Usually by the time they get to our program, yes. Most insurance programs have approved weight loss surgery for patients with body mass indexes (BMIs – estimated measurements of body fat based on height and weight) of 35 and above *if* you have co-morbidities (conditions associated with obesity), or 40 if healthy, because the surgical risks are so low and the benefit so high. So if your BMI is 35 and you're already diabetic, then losing fifty pounds would correct it better in the long term than medication, meaning your blood sugar would be under better control with weight loss than if you took a pill every day. The safety of these operations coupled with the long-term benefits make the equation different than what it was more than thirty years ago when the guidelines were first developed.

All these surgeries, all of these options to provide weight loss *invasively*, as they are called, are in evolution. The basic concepts are there, but we're always looking for a better and simpler way to achieve the results. It's always going to be a combination of several different strategies, including eating properly, exercise and surgery, that allows some sort of reduced natural eating. There will be new operations, new devices -- that will change with time -- but what we have available today are safe, time-proven options.

Are there are people who come in to see you who are too heavy for weight loss surgery?

Yes. We've done surgery on patients who are extremely large, some over 600 pounds, We know that the more people weigh, the higher the risk of complications, so if we can get some weight off that person ahead of time, we're going to try to do that. And if it means delaying surgery for six months, it doesn't mean that their journey has been delayed, it just means that when surgery does take place, it will be with less risk. So for people with a body mass index over 50, we try to get them to lose some portion of the weight ahead of time because that's going to make it safer for the patient, and easier for the surgeon who has to deal with the amount of fat surrounding the organs as well as compensate for the limitations of the laparoscopic equipment.

Most people can lose weight with a diet, but they get frustrated because they know the likelihood is that it's just going to come right back on. So if we put them through a medically-supervised weight loss program, let them know they're going to diet, lose fifty pounds and then get their surgery, and *continue* losing weight, they don't feel as if they've been cheated or put through something that's without good cause. They know that we're trying to downsize their risk by getting them to lose some weight before going into the OR. Unfortunately, it's no longer uncommon to see these people who are super morbidly obese.

What do you think inhibits weight loss the most?

If you're diabetic and on insulin, one of the side effects is that it can make you hungry and gain weight. And some of the oral medications that are used to control your blood sugars have a similar effect, so diabetics have a heck of a time losing weight. But also, as we get older, we're all usually less active. Our jobs are less active, we don't do as much physical activity, and there's the aging process itself which replaces lean muscle mass with more fat. All of these things conspire to force us to eat less just to maintain our weight. And a lot of the foods that we can't really afford to eat anymore taste good, may be higher in fat and sugar and have more calories.

You'll also see the same type of effect when you eat fast food – it's plentiful and cheap, and usually loaded with fat and calories. It's hard to eat healthy if you're on a limited budget, so it's easy to gain weight. But think about this…an estimated $2500 per year is saved on food costs for patients who have weight loss surgery.

Everyone has to work hard to keep the weight off. Genetic predisposition certainly plays a role, as does how fast you burn calories. But if you choose the surgical route, we also want to learn about your particular appetite because your urge to eat is controlled not by the stomach, but the brain. So essentially, what we're really trying to accomplish is brain surgery by operating on the stomach!

Do diabetic medications cause weight gain or keep weight on?

It doesn't take a lot of extra calories to maintain or gain weight, so many of these medications definitely make it almost impossible for diabetics to lose weight, even though they're trying as hard as they can. It's one of the reasons that weight loss surgery became legitimate, because once the relationship between being overweight and being diabetic was well established, and once we saw the epidemic of obesity in this country coincide with the epidemic of diabetes, that's when these operations were seen as tipping the balance toward the benefit. When being overweight just meant people were unhappy with their appearance or uncomfortable sitting in a chair or airplane seat or were short of breath when they climbed the stairs, it was no big deal. When people became diabetic and began dying of heart attacks and losing limbs and having strokes and losing their kidneys, all of a sudden obesity became a "real" disease and surgery became a legitimate "cure."

Now some of the medications designed to treat diabetes may actually promote weight loss and have been marketed to do both. Many of these newer drugs mimic the hormones that are changed with surgery. Unfortunately, however, most of these drugs are very expensive, and patients would have to take them their entire lives.

Do these surgeries cure diabetes? If weight is regained, can it come back?

It is essential to note that at this writing, there is no "cure" for diabetes, but at present, gastric bypass and the gastric sleeve are the surgical procedures that, collectively, are now considered to be an effective and durable "treatment" for diabetes Rather than a cure, most endocrinologists refer to the resolution of diabetes immediately following weight loss surgery as *remission*. The truth is many patients feel it is a "cure" because they are often liberated from their medications and their blood sugars return to non-diabetic levels.

While we don't know how long a remission weight loss patients will enjoy – we don't know if will last ten years or fifteen years or a lifetime – we do know that having an improvement over an extended period of time will result in less damage to their organs. More than likely it will be longstanding remission *unless the weight is regained*. If the weight loss is maintained, however, most patients can expect to halt the progression of diabetes-related disease.

So, would you say that "time is of the essence" when it comes to diabetics and weight loss surgery?

Yes. That's why being vigilant about our health – lowering our salt intake and getting our blood pressure under control, taking medicines to fix our cholesterol – is so important. Even without a "cure" per se, what we are definitely doing is slowing down that disease and preventing its progression. We all know people who have had heart attacks with normal cholesterol and diabetes and no hypertension, so the diseases can still happen, but with surgery, we're definitely taking out the component that would be contributed to by diabetes.

Is reversing diabetes the biggest benefit of surgery? What about heart disease or hypertension?

Yes to all of the above. The big ticket items are heart disease, hypertension, elevated lipids, (cholesterol), diabetes and sleep apnea, but they all work in concert to destroy your whole body. However, diabetes and heart disease are the big two. Even things like cancer have much higher rates in people who are overweight than people who are not, so that's why if you look closely, obesity causes head-to-toe problems with the body. The body's just not built to handle this extra weight, which just sort of bogs everything down.

What's the average age of people who have surgery?

Forty. And 80 percent of them are women. Usually with a couple of kids, after their forty-plus birthday, realizing that all of a sudden, they just can't keep up. They may have taken weight off after the first baby, put on more with the second and couldn't get it off. Now it's impossible. They're usually much more sensible about asking for help, not seeing it as a failure. They say *there's help out there, I can access it, I should do that.* For men, it's often perceived as a sign of weakness to ask for help, so they're usually in more dire straits before they come in. A guy will come in if his back is out or he's had a heart attack. Or he needs a knee replacement and the doctor said he'll do it if he loses fifty to a hundred pounds. When they find they can't do that by themselves, men will start thinking about asking for help.

Do you get people who come in just for cosmetic reasons?

Yes we do. Most of the time it's the younger patients, in their early twenties. However, even some of the adolescents we see can be looking at health problems. They can be seventeen years old and already diabetic or hypertensive, but their health doesn't concern them as much. They still feel invincible, and it's primarily cosmetic or social reasons that they're coming in at this point. It's funny, but the people who come in strictly for cosmetic reasons are usually relatively thin, by comparison. They'll be maybe twenty pounds overweight and want a procedure just because they've see a message on a billboard – *permanent weight loss* – along with a picture of someone who is not that heavy, so they'll think *well, they're not much bigger than I am so this should be a piece of cake for me.* They see it sometimes as preventative rather than curative, you know, just an easy way not to think about it.

People are looking for a quick fix, and these days, there are plenty of plastic surgeons selling it as a cosmetic procedure. They do balloons, liposuction, face lifts, thigh lifts, all under one roof. It's a spa package. One-stop shopping. Not what you'll find at a major medical center.

What would make you say no to a patient seeking surgery?

We often say *no*…or at least *not yet*. In our program at Cedars-Sinai, we have a rather extensive psychological and dietary assessment process where we determine if people will be able to comply with all the changes they'll have to make and be willing to deal with those disruptions in their lives. If we tell them that after surgery they can no longer eat certain foods and that the quantity of food will be limited, and it's determined that their psyche would be so disrupted by that, then we have to say that surgery is not for them *today*. They have to sort out all those personal issues first. If they're not willing to make the appropriate food choices, if they say *I'm going to eat whatever goes down, the sleeve or the bypass is going to do all the work* and they're honestly saying that that's how they're going to behave, then giving them surgery today is not in their best interest. Getting them to realize that they have to change those things in order to be successful might mean working with them for six months or so but then they'll do much better.

We're talking about a lifetime of change, not just getting the weight off and going back to the old way of life. So it's the lack of the psycho-social ability to comply and willingness to comply that kicks people out.

Physically, we test your heart and lungs, and as long as you can get through an operation, then you can be a candidate. We want people to do well with surgery, but if they're not willing to work *with* it, and they're going to hurt themselves with it, or frustrate themselves more with it, then surgery *today* is not the best thing for them. They'll need to work on those issues and opt for surgery a few months later. Otherwise, they're getting all the risks of surgery without the benefits.

What about people with eating disorders? How do you advise them?

If they have a history of anorexia and are eating next to nothing, they have to become stable and have a therapist determine that they are under control and not at risk before we give them an operation. If they're bulimic – and often a bulimic can be overweight – then they have to be psychologically stable and the eating specialist also has to feel that they are not susceptible to relapse. So any sort of inpatient mental health issue has to be dealt with. That's why we have the psycho-social evaluation, and while we don't spot it 100 percent of the time, if we discover a history, it means that we're going to spend a lot more time making sure that it's really under control. If they have surgery and do suffer a relapse, we give them extra help. Most people don't want to admit they may have an eating disorder, so if we see signs of it, we definitely have to address it.

There have been news stories about people who intentionally gain weight in order to qualify for surgery -- one woman gained 85 pounds. What would you have said?

I would have said *NO!* If she gained that much weight in order to get that operation, first of all, she didn't need it, and secondly, it sounds like there are some psychological issues that definitely need to be addressed. Having surgery can't be the only way she had to achieve her goal.

Do many people need other procedures before they come in for weight loss surgery?

Most don't, but for something like weight loss surgery, which is still thought of as elective, we have the time to make sure that it's very safe. We do all the pre-operative testing to make it safer still, so the majority of people will get through the surgery fine, no matter what. We don't want even one person to have a bad outcome that could have been avoided. For example, we would rather find out before surgery that a patient would benefit from an angioplasty and stent than after a heart attack caused by the stress of surgery. We just don't let that happen.

We occasionally see cirrhosis (liver disease) that hadn't been previously diagnosed, but most of the time it doesn't stop us from doing surgery unless it is very far advanced. Most of the time, our patients are examined so thoroughly before surgery that we don't get too many unhappy surprises when we go in.

Do you find a lot of people go through surgery and then don't comply with the post-surgical program?

I'd say if you have a good program where you have surgery, you don't find a lot of people who fall into that category. There are people, of course, who want what they want and they'll tell us what they think we want to hear, which is *yeah, I'm committed, I'll do it,* but when they find they have to work hard, it's a different story. That's one reason we worry about people who choose the clinics you see advertised on billboards and bus placards for sleeve gastrectomy surgeries. If they walk in today and have surgery tomorrow, they tend not to do so well. They don't understand the commitment it takes to make it work, so you'll see a lot more failures at programs that give it to everyone who qualifies – if they have a good, positive wallet biopsy, as they sometimes refer to patients with greater means. The truth is that some people have turned medicine into a business where the main driving force is profit rather than morality. While nobody said medicine should be a nonprofit profession, it is still important to remember that we should be helping people.

Physicians and facilities should be compensated fairly and charge fairly, but the driving force should be that we are improving patients' health or giving them a good opportunity to improve their own health.

And that's not what people find if they just go to places where they really don't understand the disease or care to understand the disease. *Head 'em up, move 'em out.* They just do the operation and they really don't teach the patient how to manage it or be committed to managing it. *Good luck, don't let the door hit you in the behind on the way out.* It's unfortunate, because if people are given a tool that could work for them and they don't understand how to use it, it won't work. If we can educate them at the beginning, we have the best chance to help them change their behaviors. If we try to salvage it later, they tend not to do as well.

*Every week seems to bring
a new "discovery." First, fat
is the culprit. Next, it's the
carbs. Which is it?*

Hey, it's BOTH. While we would like to say that, well, at
least it's not *protein* you have to avoid, the truth is that *any*
overeating will give you too many calories, so too much of
ANYTHING is no good. That's not going to get you there.

We always hear that when it comes to losing weight, slow is better. Why is that?

When you lose weight, you want to lose fat, you don't want to lose muscle or lean body mass, as we call it. And if your body goes into starvation mode as a result of an extreme diet, studies have shown that you start to break down the lean body mass. So at the end of six months, you lose more weight, but you're losing the wrong weight, and that doesn't make you healthier. What you're trying to do is keep your muscle, lose your fat and change the ratios of fat to muscle or lean body mass as you lose weight. Just being lighter isn't necessarily better.

Then what about the rapid weight loss of weight loss surgery? I've seen people who seem to disappear before my eyes.

You have to try much harder with the rapid weight loss of sleeve and bypass to get all the appropriate nutrients, so one of the things we tell everyone is that you have to get your protein in first. That means if you're not supplementing with all the liquid protein drinks that are low fat and low carbs, you've got to eat sufficient protein or you will definitely lose muscle. Heavier people, because they have to carry around extra weight, are generally very strong, so they have extra muscle and that burns calories more efficiently. But if you don't supply the proper nutrients to the muscles, then you're definitely going to get malnourished as you get thinner, and you'll have low protein storage which will make you more subject to infections and all sorts of diseases that we combat daily. That's why it's so important to lose weight in a healthy way.

What do you think about weight loss reality shows and infomercials we see on television?

The biggest problem with them is that they reinforce society's mistaken belief that all you have to do is diet and exercise and you'll keep all this weight off forever. It's like any diet. They can follow a strenuous program and lose tons of weight, but if you look at many of them a year later, most of the weight is back on.

Appropriate food selection and exercise in order to burn calories – whether it's dancing or walking around the mall or working out – coupled with the surgery (for those who choose to have it) are going to give you longstanding, durable results. Everything they're doing on TV is great to augment weight loss, but that life is not *real life* and that level of work can't be sustained. What we're looking at is a total – and permanent – change in lifestyle.

There have been some stories on the news about patients who have died from these surgeries. Just how serious is the risk?

The death rate from bariatric surgery is somewhere between one in 1000 and one in 2000, depending on who you ask, and is usually associated with *deep venous thrombosis* (DVT) or clots in the legs, *pulmonary embolisms* (blood clots in the lung), or some sort of heart condition. These are people who come in with serious problems to begin with, usually diabetic and/or hypertensive, with varying degrees of accompanying pre-existing illness. So someone between age twenty-five and forty in relatively good health, which describes the average patient who's going to be getting surgery, is at very, very low risk for ever having a problem in a reputable facility. While some procedures are being done in small, out-patient surgical centers, there are good reasons to choose a program that can admit you to the hospital overnight, especially for people who have significant sleep apnea or any other conditions that make them high risk for anesthesia. While some of the younger people are ready to rock 'n roll right after surgery, most of my patients feel much better after having spent the night in the hospital under close observation.

Bypass and sleeves are about ten times riskier than bands,

but now that we have Accredited Centers in the surgical field, they are very safe operations, on a par with having your gall bladder removed, *if* you go to a larger medical center. If you choose a small hospital or a place that does very few of these surgeries, the risk goes up considerably.

There is risk inherent in *all* surgery. I strongly urge *everyone* who is considering any of the weight loss surgeries to discuss the risks with their physicians who will help them assess the surgical risks vs. the potential health benefits.

Since many surgeons are not thought of as the warm and fuzzy variety, how important is the doctor-patient relationship in weight loss surgery?

I think that it's important even at the initial consultation that the person who's going to do your surgery actually listens to you and tries to work with you in terms of what option would be best for you. So I think that when you start out in your search, go to a surgeon who offers more than one option because that could be the only tool in the box. However, if the surgeon offers a choice between gastric bypass or the sleeve gastrectomy, and may even do the balloon and an occasional lap band, then you are more likely to be fit with something that is going to accommodate your individual needs. So I think that is your first step.

The second step is to take a look at the practice as a whole. You're going to have to be with the practice, not just with the surgeon, over the long term, and many times the relationships are stronger between the patient and nurse practitioners, dieticians and the other staff in the office, so you want to make sure the office is friendly. You're going to be involved with that office, hopefully, for the rest of your life in some way or another, so you want to make sure you're as comfortable as you can be. It's not unreasonable to shop around and keep looking until you find the right fit for you. I think that most physicians today aren't threatened by that, and if they are, then you should think twice about them. My personal opinion about that is if they do object, they're probably insecure about their own abilities and they're afraid of your going somewhere else and getting another opinion.

My patients tell me over and over that this surgery is a really big deal for them on so many levels. It's not just *I have a health problem and I'm going to get it fixed,* this is a lifestyle change, soup to nuts, for the rest of your life, so your choice deserves careful consideration.

What do you think is the biggest misconception that people come in with?

That the surgery is going to do all the work and they don't have to try hard. A lot of patients come in apologetic for needing surgery, but they shouldn't, any more than they should apologize for being diabetic or any other factors that may have contributed to their weight gain. They really can't solve it without our help and many are still blaming themselves. While we can use that guilt to change behaviors – a little bit of guilt goes a long way – you don't want to be paralyzed with it. So the biggest misconception is that having surgery is taking the easy way out. We just hope to give your brain enough help for *you* to make the right choices, to help you do the work.

In other words, surgery will give you a souped-up engine, but you still have to drive the car.

What should we be looking for in a surgical weight loss program?

I think to lose the weight safely with a surgical option requires first of all that you be ready for major surgery. You want to make sure you're healthy enough, so anything that needs to be optimized can be optimized. That's why we check out your heart and we check out your lungs and all that kind of obvious stuff, but we also have to check out your head, so that you understand what you're getting into. These are permanent changes, *lifelong* changes that you have to make, and if you're not ready or able for any reason to make those changes, then surgery is not right for you *today*.

Most people are coping with a lot of stress in their lives with regard to food, and if you can't cope with food now, you could have real issues after surgery. Food may become difficult to eat. It may make you uncomfortable if you try to eat things like ice cream after a bypass. It makes you feel sick, it's no longer your friend nor can it be your friend in that way. So there can be a mourning period or even depression following surgery. The program you choose should have the ability to identify those problems and help you find solutions, whether it be short-term medications, counseling, or just even support groups so that you don't feel like *I'm the only one experiencing this, what's wrong with me?*...as well as when things change a year or so down the line...*now I have new problems...I've lost the weight but my life's not perfect, and I thought it would be perfect if I lost the weight. Am I the only one who's feeling this way?* Then you forget where you were, meaning *I was on insulin, I could barely get out of bed, I was short of breath walking a flight of stairs.* A year later, it's infinitely better, but now you're saying *was this worth it? I just threw up my lunch again!* You forget what it was like before, so for all of those things, you need a program that's going to be there from the beginning through the, well, we never say *the end* because you're living with this forever, and offers all the support you need along the way. If you're going to have a program that offers surgery only, then they don't properly prepare you for the changes you're going to have to make and they don't properly support you afterwards with all the changes you're going to have to go through. You can find some of these things online, and you can talk to friends but you need someone to gauge what's OK and what is not.

In terms of our own program, I have my own wish list. For example, it would be great to have a gym that was attached to the program with an exercise physiologist and infinite access, more access to the dieticians for personal counseling, and things that some people find valuable, like more classes and chefs who come in and demonstrate a variety of healthy recipes...all those things would make the program even more robust.

There are two avenues to take when looking for a program. If your physician is supportive, that is always the best way to start. If you don't consult with him, if you go around him, he'll be hurt, and probably PO'd, that you've cut him out of the loop. This is a major health choice, so you shouldn't even consider cutting out your primary health care provider.

However, if he is not supportive and is unlikely to be open-minded about it, if his opinion is that surgery is a sham, that there's no benefit to surgery, that you should do this with a diet and if you can't, then there's something wrong with you, then your choice may be to cut him out of the equation while you start this journey. Try to find a new internist, one who will work *with* us in caring for you. My thought is that we don't want to take over your entire healthcare. We want to work with all the people who have been taking care of you for a long time. It's not as if you have to give them up to come see us. It's not either/or.

What do you want your new patients to know when they walk out of your office for the first time?

Most people already have an idea of what weight loss surgery is, so what I want them to know is that there is help for them, even though they've failed at every other past attempt at weight loss. I want them to know that it's not the easy fix, and I want them to not feel guilty about taking this route that's going to give them better health. I want them to realize that we're there to help and we're committed to being there for the long term, that they don't have to go through this alone. So I think they need to walk out feeling that their concerns are legitimate, that they're not crazy for seeking surgery to help fix this, that improving their health is a worthwhile endeavor and that they shouldn't feel guilty about using this option to help them get there.

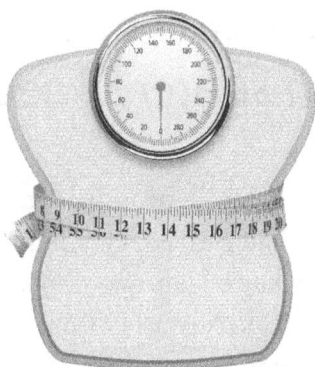

Nuts & Bolts...

Which surgery to have or, indeed, whether to have surgery at all, will be a decision you will reach with your primary physician, your surgeon and your family. Making an informed decision is a daunting task as a ton of information flies at you fast and furious. Take all the time you need to decide, ask as many questions as you like. Here are a few things I discuss with my patients along the way. I hope you find them helpful.

How do I decide which surgery I need?

A lot of times, if patients know someone who has had a particular surgery and had success, they'll gravitate toward that procedure. If they know someone who has struggled with a procedure, they'll tend to stay away from it. I think that in general we want to find the simplest way to get us there, and that's why the band was so seductive in its day. It gained popularity due to the fact that it's a very safe procedure that could result in the weight loss needed to get the co-morbidity resolution – the obesity-related health issues – and it's a fast recovery. It's hard for a lot of people with busy lives to take three weeks off from work to recover from major surgery. Back when the band was at the height of its popularity, theoretically you could have surgery on Friday and, if you had a desk job, you could be back to work on Monday and do it safely. And that's what everyone wanted.

On the other hand, gastric bypass and the sleeve gastrectomy comprise about 95% -- or more -- of the weight loss procedures we do these days because so many people say *if I'm going to do something as drastic as have surgery, it had better work, so just give me the gold standard, give me the biggest gun you have to attack this problem. If I fail with surgery, even though I know there's another potential surgery out there, I'll never be able to live with myself.* There's a lot of embarrassment in having to come to a surgeon. People are not just asking for help, they often think they've failed in what everyone thinks should work for them, which is an endless cycle of dieting and trying hard. They may think *if I fail with the surgery, that makes me an even worse person.* They tell me, *just give me the biggest thing you're willing to try. Let's get this done. Give me the biggest gun. I have to lose weight. I can't fail.* They just want the biggest, *baddest* one.

Do you give patients the surgical choices and make a recommendation?

I try to work with them, see what their expectations are, what their goals are, what their limitations are. For example, if someone is a severe diabetic, some of the features of the bypass are better at improving the health of adult-onset, insulin-dependent diabetics. If you're on a heavy dose of insulin but weren't as a child, the likelihood is that your pancreas actually does work a little bit, and the bypass is going to be better at fixing your diabetes. So I would really try to encourage you to go for that. However, if you're just on a little bit of insulin and/ or you're taking oral meds, most of the time just weight loss is going to normalize a lot of your problems. If you've been on insulin a long time, it is very difficult to get off. If you've just been on it a short time, then often just the weight loss is going to be enough to get rid of the insulin and most of the oral medications. Now if your pancreas is burned out because you waited too long to correct the problem, then you really do need the stronger operation. And while there are no guarantees, about 85 % of the people have either resolution or significant reduction in their medication after a bypass or sleeve.

How do the results differ between surgeries in terms of what would be considered success?

When all is said and done, there's probably a 20%-30% net difference overall between band and bypass. Sleeve is somewhere in between, in terms of total weight loss. I think where people get confused is that right after surgery, patients get excited to start their new lives. You look at bypass patients six months after surgery and they'll be completely into the new lifestyle, operating on autopilot, losing weight rapidly, and they just look phenomenal. However, if they don't maintain those habits five or so years out, you'll see them start to put that weight back on.

The band, with its varying degrees of restriction, offers less predictable results during those same post-surgical months. We know that it's not the instant fix that the other surgeries seem to provide and reliable data is not always available for the long term.

Fifteen years out, most people with the bypass have 50% of their excess weight off, whereas during the first year and a half, many are at over 70%. With the band, it's usually more like 40%-50%, but that's enough to significantly improve one's health. The best diets usually give you about 5%-10% reduction of excess body weight, so if we can give you 40%-50%, it beats dieting alone, no matter how you look at it.

How much pain should someone expect for each of the surgeries?

Actually the pain is very manageable. However, you have to remember that everyone experiences pain differently. Some people are up almost immediately after surgery, a little sore like they had done a few dozen crunches, while other people seem paralyzed in fear. The majority of people take a little pain medication for a couple of days, and then maybe just at night so that they sleep through, but in general, it's just sore, like having done a really significant ab workout. It's about equal for sleeve and bypass, because the pain is from the abdominal wall, not internal pain.

Probably the greatest amount of pain is for patients who have hiatal hernias because the diaphragm is moved around and irritated. They can have shoulder pain and mid-back pain. Some of the mild shoulder pain people complain about is just from having the inflation of the laparoscopy… in other words, gas. Fatigue, however, is going to be much more significant with the bypass and sleeve, which might last four to six weeks. Whereas some patients – especially younger people – are back to normal within a couple of weeks, it is not unusual for others to find themselves falling asleep in their mashed potatoes.

Is there an optimum age range for surgery? How old is too old?

The primary reason for weight loss surgery is to prevent and cure disease. In order to stop the damage caused by diabetes, hypertension and the like, we look to see that the patient has a decent life expectancy ahead. So we're looking for optimum potential health benefits rather than chronological age. We wouldn't be doing surgery if someone had three months left to live, but most people who have five years or more of expected life can benefit from it and now many people are living well into their eighties. I have a healthy eighty-year-old patient who had surgery more than ten years ago – you'd never guess she was eighty! Even with older people, the benefit can be great. Losing forty or fifty pounds can make a huge difference in terms of getting around on arthritic knees or deteriorating hips. So the targets are different for these people.

Today, we're constantly hearing about economists who are running the figures to weigh costs against benefits. And with diabetics, for example, it now takes twelve to eighteen months to recoup the costs in drugs and treatment against the cost of the surgery.

So, how old is too old? I think that at the top end, patients have to be able to safely get through surgery and not have some sort of disease that's going to shorten their lives in the next year and, conservatively, have at least five years life expectancy. So that means seventy-five-year-old women are still candidates, if they're healthy.

Of course, the younger we get them as adults, the better. The earlier we can reverse disease and arrest its damage, or prevent disease altogether, the better the long-term outcome.

Some sources say gastric bypass is the most popular surgery. Others claim it's the sleeve. Which surgery do you do the most?

Depending on where you are, and this goes for a lot of procedures in medicine, one is going to outnumber the other. Right now, we do about 30% bypass and 70% sleeve gastrectomy, with the occasional lap band accounting for a very small percentage along with other available procedures.

The popularity of the sleeve can be attributed to its relative simplicity (no re-routing of intestines) and safety. It's important to note that here at Cedars-Sinai, we hold the MBSAQIP (Metabolic and Bariatric Surgery Accreditation and Quality Improvement Program) accreditation by the American College of Surgeons and the American Society for Metabolic and Bariatric Surgery, so we do a fair number of *revisional* surgeries, that is, bands, bypasses and sleeves as well as older procedures that are referred to our center to get fixed. But for first-timers, it's sleeve, bypass and band, in that order. Some practices don't offer all of these options, so their numbers will vary, even 90%-100% sleeve, with no revisions.

People generally go elsewhere to have those surgeries fixed so many surgical centers may deny there's even a problem, which reinforces the idea of staying away from choosing facilities you see advertised on a billboard or the side of a bus.

In fact, we can't say often enough to get a trusted referral -- or two -- from your primary care physician, preferably at a major accredited hospital or medical center. These are not procedures where you want to cut corners. And now that obesity has been designated as a disease, more and more insurance companies are covering bariatric surgery. There are in excess of 250,000 weight loss surgeries performed in the U.S. each year, and that number will increase as insurance coverage becomes more and more prevalent.

What is sleep apnea and what does it have to do with weight loss surgery?

Sleep apnea is when all the soft tissue at the back of the throat collapses when you sleep and it blocks the airway because it's too heavy and soft, and so you obstruct, then you stop breathing (apnea). Finally, after your brain is starving for oxygen, you wake up, even if you don't remember awakening each time it happens. When patients tell me they snore and don't sleep through the night, I pretty much know they have sleep apnea. Most of our patients have some degree of sleep apnea when they go into surgery. The best treatment for them would be to lose weight. So as long we are watching them when they are in the hospital and not sending them home immediately, we can keep them safe. If someone has been diagnosed with *severe* sleep apnea and has surgery in a surgical center and is sent home the same day after anesthetics, then it can be a problem. Narcotics or anesthetics, pain medicines or sedatives used to put you out for the surgery all blunt the ability to wake up, so for those with severe apnea, it's a riskier proposition.

I've heard a lot of patients have hiatal hernias. What are they?

A hernia is when something pushes through a hole that it's not supposed to push through. The *hiatus* is a hole in the diaphragm, an opening at the very top of the stomach where it meets the esophagus. The chest and the abdomen are separated by the diaphragm. In order for things to go from the mouth into the abdomen, there has to be an opening for the esophagus to pass through. If it's wide or gets enlarged, then the top of the stomach can slide up into the chest.

That's a hiatal hernia. We see them a lot in overweight patients and we routinely fix them when we get in there.

Why are you asking people to go on a low-calorie diet for two weeks before surgery?

We do that for all patients – regardless of the operation they choose. There are some studies out there that show that rapid weight loss or low calorie diets for a period of a week or two, or even three, prior to surgery helps shrink the liver. The visceral fat – or fat that's in the organs – gets dissolved or used as you fast, and studies have shown that livers swollen and big with fat shrink after a short time on a low-calorie liquid diet. That gives us more space to work – and more than that, when the liver is swollen with fat, it's softer and easier to fracture, which can lead to bleeding. So not only can it get in our way it can lead to complications, which is why we decided to start the diet two weeks ahead. We chose two weeks, because if we asked for three weeks before surgery and then two weeks after, it might be too much for many patients to comply. The liquid diet has to do with the size of the liver and the surrounding fat, and because men especially carry most of their fat around their organs, rather than on their thighs or other places, getting that to melt away gives us more space.

There's a lot to move around in there and a lot of things to find, so we would rather you didn't go out for a Last Supper before surgery, though I'm sure a lot of people do. They're just smart enough not to tell us. What we do is to check their weight throughout their pre-operative evaluation period and if someone puts on a significant amount of weight, then we wind up canceling the surgery. We tell them that up front, because a lot of people will treat it as their last chance to party, but we're aware that there is still a lot of information we never hear about.

What am I going to have to give up? And how do those things differ with each surgery?

While it differs a little bit with each operation -- and each person -- what you have to give up is eating large portions and doing so at unregulated speed. That's for sure. You just can't do it. If you try to do it, you're going to be awfully uncomfortable. You also have to give up things that are going to sabotage you, so carbohydrates that are liquid and fatty foods have to be extremely limited because these things greatly inhibit weight loss.

With the bypass and, to a lesser extent, the sleeve, people can get an adverse reaction to the wrong foods called *dumping* that's really unpleasant. It kind of feels like a cross between low blood sugar and a panic attack. Sometimes with cramping, vomiting and diarrhea. Altogether an unpleasant experience. And while each episode passes fairly quickly, patients can experience dumping for the first couple of years after surgery. So you're giving up ice cream and cookies and cakes and candies. A lot of people really enjoy those things, but they're making the choice to be healthier and they know that anything more than a taste here and there is going to result in real discomfort.

There will be foods that can be difficult to eat for the foreseeable future, but these things differ for different people. You can pretty much forget about eating bread in a sandwich. If you took sourdough bread, sliced it really thin and toasted it, that's crunchy and less likely to get stuck, but eating a piece of bread? Not such a good idea. I got a call from a patient who had been in bed all weekend from pain caused by one bite of a King's Hawaiian roll. That won't be on her menu again anytime soon.

Anything that's gummy and sticky, like sushi rice, will plug up that small opening we leave you. Anything with a lot of gluten, if they haven't put a lot of fat in it to make it slippery, then it's going to clog it up, so you have to give up those things. But for the most part, you'll be able to find foods you can eat – and specific things that work for you. For example, Akmak crackers are crunchy and they can be carbohydrates you can use, so not all bread products will be gone. There's just going to be a much smaller group that you'll be able to tolerate.

Do I have to give up these things forever?

If you want to maintain the weight loss forever, yes. Although early on, if the only reason you weren't eating those foods is because you felt crummy and you just started adding ice cream again two years later, you'll find you can definitely get a lot of ice cream down. You have to make a long-term commitment to stay away from those concentrated calories. And the other thing you have to give up to a large extent is the freedom to eat with abandon, because even though you're free from the weight, you still have to structure your life a little bit more so that you can make healthy choices for yourself every day. You have to make a list of where you can get healthy foods or you have to prepare a little bit more and bring them with you, because if you skip a bunch of meals, you're going to be hungry, you'll eat too fast and make yourself uncomfortable. Remember, the vending machines have bad choices, the *roach coach* has bad choices, all those places we get fast foods. You'll find yourself wanting to eat more healthfully because being free of that extra weight feels so much better.

What is sliming, and should I have a wastebasket ready when I read this answer?

Sliming is what often occurs if food gets stuck. You block off the opening, or that doorway out of that little stomach. Since your body is constantly making saliva to lubricate things, that slime is all that saliva piling up on top. You reach a threshold, it comes back on you and it's pushing in both directions. The offending item gets pushed down, but the slime comes up, so that the blockage is gone but you receive the gift of slime.

The restrictions we create vary by the person and the procedure, but sliming can happen with all of the operations. A big hunk of meat can block up a sleeve, it can block up a bypass, it can block up a band, so your body's response is extra salivation to try to lubricate the way down.

A little gross, but a good reminder to chew, chew, chew. It will all become second-nature pretty quickly.

I've gone through three months with virtually no weight loss. However, my face is thinner and my clothes are bigger. What gives?

The body is always remodeling. Over and over. Lean muscle has replaced fat, so if you are building muscle and losing fat, you can be the same weight but actually smaller. And *younger*. So ask yourself, *how do I feel?* If the answer is *great*, don't worry!

Why do you stop losing weight at any given point?

Simply put, the body defends its set point. The brain has a set point of weight and what the operations allow you to do is move that set point to a new level, but not usually to the ideal weight as dictated by the insurance tables. Your body has created this set point of where IT thinks it needs to be and in order to convince it otherwise, you have to voluntarily reduce caloric intake or do things that are going to make your body burn calories more efficiently, like exercising to produce more lean body mass. Now, what we'd like to see in the future would be the development of drugs that would allow you to do both of those things – change the set point even further or burn more calories – and do it safely rather than taking speed (amphetamines) like so many people did in the past.

It also appears that genetics plays a role. One day soon, we should be able to do one of those well-advertised genetic tests to determine how well a patient would do with each type of surgery. We are making similar strides in treating cancer, where genetics predicts response to chemotherapy.

With regard to all the surgeries, how do you know when you're done losing weight, when you've gone as far as you can go?

Usually a good rule of thumb is that at about two years, most of the operations have sort of reached maximal weight loss. However, if you've never tried to work *with* the operations, you've never really complied with the dietary regimen, and later on down the line you decide *OK, I'm serious about this now*, then that two-year period starts over. But if you've gone through the program, you've eaten the appropriate foods, you've exercised and all that, then most of the time by two years, you kind of figure out how much weight you're going to lose. With the sleeve it's about 60% of the excess weight on average, if you are provided access to good dieticians, good psychologists or social workers, and perhaps support groups. Bypass can average 70%. However, for the places where they just do the surgery, kick you out the door and don't really follow you, the results are less predictable. While the *average* losses are noted above, you're always going to find a population who doesn't do as well. They're going to say it didn't work, but the truth of the matter for many is that *they* didn't make it work. It's always a marriage between you and your procedure. You can cheat your operation if you want to, and it won't do you any good. So you have to remember to work *with* any of the operations.

With the bypass and, to a lesser extent, the sleeve, the accompanying dumping helps you to stay away from the liquid carbs and the fats, but if dumping goes away, which it does, you become less sensitive. That generally happens about the two-year mark. That's when you'll see some people gain some of the weight back. They couldn't do ice cream the first month after surgery because they'd feel really sick, but three years later, they *can* eat ice cream – and all sorts of other things – and some patients put on approximately 15% of their weight.

How much regaining of weight do you see?

The majority of people don't regain much. You're probably playing with about 15% overall, meaning if you sort of veer off the path of appropriate foods, if you're not as vigilant as when you first started, you're not going to gain all of the weight back. That's why you have to develop good habits up front, because it's easier to be committed from the outset than to break bad habits later on. Of course, there will always be those who will say *let's take this operation out for a spin and see what it can do on its own. I can always make a commitment somewhere down the line.* Problem is, you can't trade it in, so you might as well drive it carefully right off the assembly line.

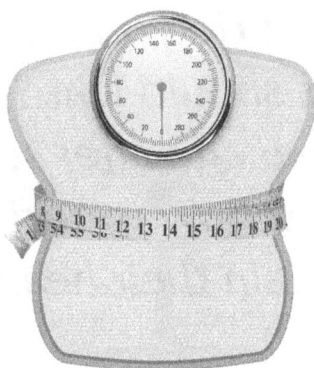

Life Changes...

If you happen to read this book in its entirety, you may notice the recurring theme that weight loss surgery carries with it certain truths...notably that it is not a quick fix and that success requires a huge commitment on your part. Your life will change, because your LIFESTYLE will change. How you eat. What you eat. Your entire relationship with food. The surgery does not "work" all by itself – YOU make it work. And this is forever. The rest of your life. So think about it carefully. The consideration of this commitment is as important as the decision to have the surgery itself. I'm a surgeon. I love doing these operations, making significant changes in people's lives. But you've got to meet me halfway, then take the ball and run with it.

What do you think patients should learn about how to manage after surgery – how to eat, how to reclaim and maintain their health?

So many of the popular diet programs find someone else planning all your meals and giving you pre-measured portions, asking you to pick one from column A, one from column B, eat them three times a day, and you're probably not learning what the nutritional content of the food is or what the proper choices are. So I think part of what you learn from a good program is a basic nutritional education, even so simplistic as saying *what is a carbohydrate, what is a fat, what is a protein. These are examples of foods that have those things in them.* Having sample diets is great, but in our society you still have to make choices. People need to learn to read labels – we stress that – so they actually know what's in the food. They're not just being handed a box and told to *eat this.* I also think that taking away hunger for a lot of people encourages them to read the labels. I mean, if you're not starving all the time and are just putting something in your mouth because you need to, you'll read the label a little more carefully and say *you know, that's not a great choice.* So I think the surgery allows you to actually think about it, whereas before you weren't thinking, you were on autopilot and just consuming.

So much eating *is* done on autopilot. *Because it's 7 o'clock and time to eat. Because I'm watching American Idol. Because the game's on and there's that Doritos commercial again.* Unfortunately, we do have a lot of social expectations that have been developed or culturally passed down to us. So someone may be telling you when you should eat breakfast, lunch and dinner, or someone says *you should be hungry at 6 o'clock because that's when I'm making dinner, and you need to eat a full plate, you're wasting food, people are starving in Ethiopia.* And I think that we're also eating out a lot. In restaurants, we're given portions that are meant to feed multiple people rather than a single person, and we've come to think that's what we're supposed to eat. When people get serious about this process, I think they learn that the portion sizes needed to maintain their weight are much smaller than they ever imagined.

We sometimes run into family members who say *she's not eating enough!* We say *well, we checked her labs and she's nutritionally replete, meaning her protein levels are all great, her vitamin levels are all great, she's maintaining a healthy weight so she's eating enough, you just THINK she needs to eat more.* And that's *their* problem. It may be a cultural thing since in a lot of cultures, food is love. *If you don't eat my food, you don't love me.* If somebody comes over, it's welcoming, and you can't let anyone go hungry, so you make enough for the Fifth Army.

I think for a lot of people satisfying hunger is different from feeling stuffed, but a lot of people think they should feel stuffed after every meal and they're not going to get that

feeling unless they overeat greatly. While some people think
it's not Thanksgiving unless they have to unbutton their pants
afterwards, some people are doing that after every meal.

So, how much do you have to know about proper nutrition?
A lot! The more you know, the better choices you will make,
the more variety you will discover and the greater your success
following surgery. (My own patients report that their newfound
knowledge of nutrition has made their entire families better
eaters. *They* may be surprised…but *I'm* not!)

How important do you think it is to have realistic expectations?

I think that's the most important thing. If you don't have realistic expectations about how you're going to have to eat or how you're going to have to change your life, you probably won't succeed. If you think the only thing that's important is to be as thin as a Vogue model, then you're setting yourself up for disappointment. If you're only going to be satisfied with 100 percent excess weight loss and you get 50 percent, you may tend to view that as a failure and you're more likely to quit your good behavior. If you think the operation's going to do all the work and you have to do nothing, then you probably won't stick to an exercise regimen. Unless you're already an exercise fanatic, it's tough to adopt an exercise lifestyle, especially if you believe it isn't needed. So setting up the expectation of what surgery will do for *you* is the important thing. First of all, you have to work with it, it's a lot of hard work, and it's not a perfect solution. Success requires a lot of effort on your part, and everyone's a little bit different, so you shouldn't give up if you don't get 100 percent of the results that you want. Just because the guy next to you is doing well, that doesn't mean that he is working somehow harder than you are.

How important is the support of people you live with?

It's very important. There are going to be difficult days.
You have to change your eating habits. If people are always
being critical of you, maybe even criticizing the benefit of
what you achieved, many people aren't self-confident enough
not to listen. So some people who will help you not eat that
extra cookie, or encourage you not to even bring them into
the house, or maybe even not eat them themselves, that's
important. For people not to diminish your accomplishments
and to be supportive is much more beneficial. If you need to
exercise and you have someone to do that with, that's all going
to be positive.

We've seen that relationships are often codependent and
someone with weight issues may also lack self-confidence or
feel like she's settling and can't do any better. As she loses
weight, her self-image will improve and if her mate is insecure,
he may sabotage her efforts because all of a sudden his partner
is losing weight, feeling more attractive, feeling more self-
confident, and getting attention she didn't get before. And
sometimes the patient will say *hey, I really didn't like this guy too
much anyway and I can do better,* so there's additional disruption
in the dynamic. That's why support is always very important and
why patients should take advantage of support groups… having
people to share things with, positive and negative.

People react differently to substantial weight loss. While most people like the attention and enjoy feeling better and looking better, there will always be those who will think *I'm still a fat person in a skinny person's body*. That body image doesn't change along with the reality when they look in the mirror.

Society makes overweight people feel like they are failures. It's part of that whole discrimination thing we have to get rid of. There are the health-related problems, the heart disease and diabetes that we focus on getting rid of, but we also need to address the societal problem that everyone thinks being overweight is some kind of moral or character weakness. If there are two people of equal qualification applying for the same job, let me tell you that the thin one's going to get it. Weight is sort of the last area where discrimination is sanctioned.

What do you tell people about giving up their lifelong habits... all the things that add up to a huge lifestyle change?

The people we do best with, the ones we can help the most, are the ones who come for medical reasons. If they're coming for strictly cosmetic benefits of weight loss, then it's harder to convince them to give up things in their lives. Most people come in because they have diabetes or high blood pressure or they've had a heart attack or they need to have knees or hips replaced, those kinds of things, and their health has really confronted them with a choice. And they see it as *the rest of my life is going to be continued deterioration if I continue on this course.* A lot of them will say *the party's over...or at least the decadence of the party is over and what I'm getting back is a lot more vibrancy, a lot better health, a longer, better quality for my future life.* They've had enough experience and been confronted with enough adversity that they can actually see that as a reality rather than just something they've heard or read about. We grow up hearing *if you don't brush your teeth, your teeth are going to fall out.* It's hard to visualize that when you're ten years old, but when you're forty and have had a couple of root canals, it's easier to see that it's important to do this stuff. Luckily, most of our patients have had enough life experience that they see there's give-and-take in most everything, so the majority of them are willing to give up at least a little to get the benefits.

I've always been a volume eater. Is that OK, as long as it's low-calorie, low-fat food?

Yes, if you are losing an appropriate amount of weight after surgery. If you're not losing weight, however, you're no doubt getting too many calories in. Because of the way the energy equation works, in order to lose weight, you have to take in less energy than you need to maintain that weight. Muscle tissue burns more calories than inert tissue like fat, so the more muscle you have, the more calories you'll need to maintain. The hotter your body is running, the more fuel that it's burning. Just like a hotrod, it's just sitting there burning more. So exercise helps burn calories as well as having more muscle mass burns calories. Looked at another way, some people are like a Prius rather than an SUV, so they need fewer calories. They can't just look at the person's plate next to them in a restaurant and say *she's skinny. If she can eat that much, I can eat that much.*

For our patients, since we we have greatly reduced the stomach's capacity, you'll find you'll have more control to help you shave off those extra 100 calories or 200 calories in a day without feeling deprived.. That's not much, and it will help you start losing weight again.

What is the difference between not being hungry and being full?

The magic word we use is *satiety*. And that means *satisfaction with your state*. If you aren't satisfied, then you're hungry. That's a different feeling from *I need to feel stuffed*. Ideally, you really want to stop is when *hunger* is gone, you don't want to continue eating until you feel like you've just had Thanksgiving dinner.

For a lot of people, hunger – or that insatiable desire to seek out food when your body is telling you it has to be fed – dissipates in about fifteen minutes. We try to get people to differentiate between that need to feel stuffed – what most people believe feeling full is – and when one is satisfied, that is, no longer hungry. It's one of the reasons we ask you to take a pause, take a time-out, take a break, try not to eat continuously for two hours, but stop after half an hour and let your body catch up. Many times you'll realize that you're not eating because you're hungry, you're eating because you're bored or because everybody else is eating, because it tastes good, because it's *there*. Sometimes people get so full, they're stuffed and ready to throw up, but they'll still try to stick one more bite into their mouths. It's not for hunger they're eating at that point, and that's what we try to get people to understand as they adjust to their new eating patterns.

I really enjoy food.
Big plates of delicious food.
I'm afraid I'm
really going to miss that!

You're still going to be able to enjoy food. Delicious food. Just not as much of it. You will soon learn why doggie bags were invented and you will be able to enjoy your favorites for dinner the next day and maybe even lunch the day after that. Your choices should become healthier, too, as you begin to lose weight since you won't want to sabotage your own efforts.

Food will still be delicious, but probably not as important in your life as it once was. One of my patients, whose social engagements always revolved around getting together with friends for meals, told me that her new mantra is *it's not the food, it's the company.* And while it may have taken a little getting used to, she is now enjoying herself as much as she ever did. She just makes different choices.

If portions have to be so small, how do you get out of the habit of mindless eating, like putting your hand into a bag of chips or a bowl of nuts?

One strategy is to get into the practice of measuring out those "mindless" snacks and putting them in a cup so that you actually have an end to it. It's much like when people want to establish good sleeping habits. If you put a TV in your bedroom and you jump into bed and watch TV, you might have problems with insomnia because bed now represents entertainment and there are no defined limits. Same thing is true with food. You don't want to eat the whole bag of chips, so the last thing you want to do is put the bag on your lap and mindlessly eat while you're distracting yourself with TV. You want to create a very defined place to eat, so we recommend that you sit down at the table and have a time or a structure to your eating. Plan for it to be no longer than thirty minutes. Most people are not hungry after about fifteen minutes, and then they just eat for taste or out of habit, so what you want to do is minimize the distractions when you're eating. The TV is the biggest culprit, of course, because it's easy to just put things in your mouth without thinking about it at all. You want to make eating its own activity, associated with hunger, not just eating because it's nighttime and you're relaxing. It's all a matter of keeping your head in the game, taking responsibility for what, when and where you eat, and making good choices.

It's a given that many weight loss surgery patients will be doing a certain amount of throwing up. How much is too much and what's the danger?

There are several degrees of what we define as vomiting. There's very violent vomiting which is definitely something we never want. It leads to bouts of retching, more than just regurgitation. Then there's what many people will describe as a *wet burp*, so it's very similar to what was just in their mouths, very transient...it doesn't even fly out of their mouths, they just feel the food come back up. While those kinds of episodes aren't dangerous, the violent retching episodes can lead to rupturing of the esophagus, not to mention the damage it can do to your teeth. So if it's infrequent, meaning not more than once every couple of weeks, we consider that to be well-adapted. When you're doing it daily, or even at every meal, and you're otherwise doing everything right, you need to have your surgeon check you out to make sure everything is still where he or she put it.

The bottom line is that if you're a bypass or sleeve patient who vomits with any regularity, you're probably either eating too fast or not chewing your food properly and still doing behaviors that are not perfect. So the answer is that we like to see throwing up reduced to almost never unless you are occasionally distracted when eating and make a mistake.

What about not drinking while you eat? Is it because you are able to wash down too much food?

The reason for not eating and drinking at the same time is that you want the food to maintain its texture and thickness (if it manages to stay where you put it) and if you're constantly adding liquid to the solid, you're essentially making soup. You'll rinse the food faster through your pouch, and you'll ultimately take in more calories before your brain gets the signal to stop. If the food is down there and the pouch is full and you try to take a big drink of water on top of it, you are going to overfill it and you'll be throwing up more. And people tend to swallow more with bigger gulps of liquid than they would with solid food. So while drinking during meals is a hard habit to break, it's one of the necessary "rules" we ask you to follow.

One of my patients encountered a guy who was concerned that he didn't think he could comply when it came to not drinking with meals. She told him that those are the rules. *The rules are there for a reason. If you don't want to follow the rules, don't have the surgery.* I think that was good advice. You've got to be ready to make the commitment, and it's lifelong. Motivation to adhere to all of the lifestyle changes is usually the greatest, or we hope it is, right after surgery, and so it's much easier to develop all the habits that you have to carry

through for the rest of your life to be successful if you do it at
the beginning.

No caffeine?
You're taking away my caffeine???
Are you kidding me? Why?

Well, caffeine is an appetite stimulant, for starters, and it dehydrates you, too. Some people drink a caffeinated beverage to hydrate themselves where water will do a better job of that. Also, anything that stimulates you and makes you nervous generally makes people agitated and they're going to look for something to calm themselves down. (Many people have that relationship with sugar.) The more anxious you are, the more you're going to seek out something to help, and for a lot of people who are overweight, that's going to be food. So while we advise patients to give up caffeine entirely, I've been known to negotiate one cup of coffee per day for the die-hards among us.

Why no carbonated drinks, even diet soda? Is it just a discomfort thing?

With all of these operations, we've left you with such a small stomach, the air bubbles that are the carbonation in soda can create painful gas. So it is, indeed, a discomfort thing, even after just a swallow of a carbonated drink. However, over time, it may even lead to the pouch stretching because your body tries to accommodate any sort of stress you put on it, and if you're constantly trying to blow up your stomach like a balloon, the body at some point is going to say *OK, let's make this balloon a little bit bigger so that it doesn't hurt so much.* If you try to drink regular soda, it's like adding insult to injury. It's all sugar and has a ton of calories, and it's liquid, so it's going to go through easily, and because it's going to potentially dilate your pouch, it can ruin your operation long-term. And you have to remember that even if you lose all the weight you want to lose in the first six months, you've got to live with this thing forever. It's just like your new car… if you're going to hit every pothole with it, your car's not going to last as long as it would if you would just baby it a little bit.

No ibuprofen? You haven't walked a mile with my knees!

Aspirin and ibuprofen, which can be irritating to normal stomachs and cause bleeding with continual use, can cause profound damage to the little stomach area we leave you with after surgery. There are some other drugs that would be safe to use on a limited basis, but unfortunately, even some of the non-narcotic variety have some dependency issues, so you don't want to take them every single day. You can take something when the pain is severe but you have to make sure everything's crushed and/or washed down with a lot of water so that it's going to minimize the danger of it sitting in the pouch and causing damage. What many people find, however, is that as the weight comes off, the need for the drugs lessens as the back and joint pain subside.

As the operations go, the sleeve would be the most tolerant of daily ibuprofen use. So with all things being equal, the patient with bad joint disease probably gets a sleeve.

Why does hair loss seem to be so common after surgery?

Hair loss, fingernails getting a little more brittle and skin getting drier are all very common just because as you lose weight, the body thinks it's starving. It's trying to triage resources, while trying to say *I don't need to waste my energy building hair that primarily serves to keep heat in if I don't have the resources to stay alive.* It sort of shunts all the resources to all the things that are going to be more vital, because you're going into starvation mode. If you don't eat protein, your body doesn't have a building block for hair so protein is always the number one thing you should be eating. If you don't get the vitamins needed to build hair and nails because you're eating less, then that's going to contribute also. But it's really the starvation… the body sort of shutting down, turning down the temperature on the furnace. It's shutting down what it perceives to be less vital functions, and hair is one of those things. Once, when asked if the incidence of hair loss was pretty equal between men and women, I answered that actually bald men lose less hair, but that didn't go over too well!

Biotin is one of the vitamins that helps with hair growth, so when you start to eat less, if you don't eat foods that are rich in biotin, you can experience hair loss. Most people wind up taking a vitamin with biotin that promotes bone and hair support along with making sure they consume adequate protein.

Do you feel that alcohol is a major issue with your patients?

Yes, a lot of people are used to medicating themselves with food, and alcohol is often used as a substitute to make people forget some of their problems. It's also liquid so it goes down relatively easily. And then there is something known as *transfer addiction*, so there is some risk of taking your food obsession and turning it over to another type of drug that makes you feel better, like alcohol, in many cases. If we know that someone is a problem drinker, we will send them for counseling just because we know they are at risk for becoming a bigger abuser post-operatively. One theory is that if you take two or three drinks a night, you are an abuser of alcohol and have a problem. Some people say *a bottle of wine a night? No problem. A six pack a night? No problem.* What they may not realize is that it's empty calories to begin with. First they drink their calories and then can't focus enough to pay attention to what they eat. It's a lose-lose situation – but unfortunately not in terms of excess weight.

Tell me a little more about the transfer addiction between food and alcohol.

One school of thought is that overindulging in food fills a psychological need, so it is one of the components that psychiatrists are examining while looking at addictive types of personalities. For most people who are overweight, their particular addiction is food. So if you take away the ability to get your "drug" of choice, which is food, then it's going to be easier to fall into the pattern of obsession with something else that provides a similar sort of satisfaction or escape. It might be alcohol or cigarettes or narcotics or marijuana – any or all of those things – since people are much more susceptible because they're transferring that loss of food into something else that they're finding enjoyable.

Many of the people who come through this program are addicted to food. They love food. They're wired to love food, some more than others. A lot of people are willing to trade, while some aren't. That's one of the reasons for the psycho-social evaluations we do before surgery. We look at how dependent people are and how their lives are structured, because if someone's life pretty much sucks outside of their ability to have food, it's going to be much easier to fall into the trap of another unhealthy habit. Now one of the "rules" we set up is not to drink alcohol – at least for a period of time – but some people do anyway, especially if they don't have a good support structure. We need to learn whether they have good friends and family, if they have healthy outlets or if they feel isolated, so that they don't turn to something that's there and easy and pushed at us pretty much everywhere we turn. Even people who smoked cigarettes for a long period of time can go cold turkey with those legal "drugs," but you can't with food, which makes it much harder to kick that habit.

What if I need surgery, but I still want to have children?

What we don't want is for someone to try to get pregnant while they're actively losing weight. Now with the bypass or sleeve, that weight loss period is about a year and a half before people stop. We'll say in order to make sure your body's stabilized and properly nourished, ladies, you should wait until two years after a bypass or sleeve to conceive. So if your intent is to get pregnant within the next few months, you shouldn't be having the weight loss surgery today.

However, as we all know, sometimes *life happens* and babies arrive on the scene. That's when your surgeon should be consulted to help guide you through a healthy pregnancy and weight loss following delivery.

How much do we really need to learn about proper nutrition? Isn't eating less going to be enough?

No, because like it or not, we tend to get our portion sizes from TV or the size of our plates. And, we've been taught or conditioned the wrong way, since all the fast food places entice you to have a double cheeseburger, large fries and a thirty-two-ounce Coke, and most restaurant portions are ridiculous.

I talk to a lot of people about nutrition, and I can tell you that for the most part, they sort of have general concepts of what a protein is, what a carbohydrate is, what a fat is, but in the real world, they don't know what a real portion size is, whether it's a deck of cards, or the palm of your hand, or what the building blocks of those portions are, how much fat vs. protein, and so on. So you *have* to become label readers and, at the beginning, you may even become food *weighers* until you get a good handle on it. We have to reset our brains and use any tricks we can find to teach us new ways of looking at what appropriate diets are.

After fifty years of drumming the food pyramid into the minds of American children, it has finally been abandoned for the image of a plate, with vegetables occupying the majority of the space, because the pyramid was just not working. Even

Michelle Obama became involved when she, as First Lady, advocated the use of a plate that more people can relate to, and one that reduces our portion size. It's re-educating Americans who may not learn it from Mom who equates food with love and who may not know a great deal about nutrition, nor from a super-sizing fast-food place with "value" deals. If we truly look at our eating habits, we'll find that most of the time, they're not appropriate.

Of course, that doesn't stop us from getting a chuckle from former Daily Show host Jon Stewart who reportedly wrote the following note to Chili's Restaurants: *Thank you, Chili's, for putting the calorie count of all your food on your menu. What part of "I don't give a crap" don't you understand?*

How important are vitamins, really? Shouldn't I be OK if I just eat healthy?

When we check our patients' vitamin levels, even for those who are hundreds of pounds overweight, the vitamin levels are low, despite the volume of food they consume. Since all weight loss surgery prevents you from getting enough of your vitamins to one extent or another, vitamins are going to be a non-negotiable "rule" to follow for the rest of your life. With the gastric bypass, there's an absolute requirement for vitamin supplements, the most of the three surgeries. The sleeve is also going to require vitamins, because we're taking away a majority of the stomach, part of which you need to absorb vitamins.

The majority of people make choices that aren't perfect and most people don't want to think about every morsel they eat and how to balance it, so taking that vitamin pill is an insurance policy to make sure you're getting the right amount. As long as you don't overdo it by taking mega-doses of several supplements, the body just sheds the extra that you give it. And it's something you have to do continuously, you can't just take vitamins once every six months to catch up.

For those of you who are not habitual vitamin-takers, this is one of the lifestyle changes you just *have* to make. These vitamins should be chewable or liquid since you have to take them every day for the rest of your life, and crushing vitamins and putting them into your mouth is pretty unpleasant. We don't want something that is so important to your overall health to be punitive, so shop around and find something you can tolerate.

How important is exercise, really? What if I don't?

If you don't, you're going to have to cut back your eating more than you would if you did. A lot of people will say *if I exercise, I get hungry and I eat more,* but in general, that's not the case. If you exercise, you're going to build up more muscle mass, and since lean muscle burns calories more efficiently, that's going to allow you to consume more calories and have more variety. If you really restrict yourself, and just sit there and do nothing but breathe and watch TV, then you're going to have to cut back your calories even more than that extra few hundred calories a day that you would burn during exercise.

Look at exercise as any prescription your physician would give you. You wouldn't think of not taking medication prescribed by your doctor, would you? Bottom line, don't fight it. Find something you like to do – maybe dancing or taking nature walks – and make it a part of your daily life. Our patients who do that have greater success than those who don't. They not only lose more weight, they're healthier, stronger, *younger* than those who remain sedentary. Believe me, I wish there were some magic bullet that could offer the benefits of exercise without the exertion, but there just isn't.

Don't you feel that success begets success, that is, isn't it easier to say 'no' so that you don't undo the good you have done?

Yes, that's definitely true. People are proud of what they've accomplished so it's much easier to stay on track once you've had a lot of success. However, many people tend to get complacent after a while too. They want to maintain their success but at the same time they don't want to live with the sacrifice. They want to have their cake and eat it too. Literally. And they generally do, which is why two-thirds of the population is overweight.

It doesn't help that Starbucks now offers the 31-ounce *Trenta* drinks. The 20-ounce *Venti* isn't big enough, so even those high-calorie coffee drinks are getting bigger. And of course, they'll put out the nutritional chart and people will ignore it. A patient recently complained that she reads those charts in every restaurant she goes to and it generally ruins her evening. I can't say I'm sorry that it does.

Most restaurants cater to the celebration mentality so if you just pick things that taste great without concern for the health value, you're going to wind up ordering the fattiest, highest-calorie thing nearly every single time, like starting with an appetizer which, in some places, can be 2500 calories all by itself.

They say that the best bite of a treat is the first bite, and the next best bite is the last bite. So, two bites ought to do it, don't you think? That's reasonable. That's why we talk about *lifestyle* changes. We talk about being committed to working *with* all of the operations and being committed to trying to make those changes so that you don't feel that you'll only be happy if you eat the whole thing. And most people who do make those changes realize that success is achievable that way.

*You deal with people every day
who need to lose a lot of weight
and part of your counsel is
about how to eat properly.
Has this affected the way YOU eat?*

Yes, it has definitely made me a healthier eater. It doesn't mean I don't like the same tasty foods that everyone else likes, but I definitely try to portion them out. We're designed to like things that taste fantastic and most of the time they are high-fat foods. There are very few people who don't like those appealing foods.

Personal choices I make? Zero sugar beverages. I also can't remember the last time I went to a fast food restaurant like McDonald's or Burger King, even though I love their fries. Those things I stay away from with a passion, just knowing it's healthy to do so. I also wouldn't bury my salad in mayonnaise-based salad dressings, knowing I'm just fooling myself if I do that. While we all overindulge every once in a while, we have to remember that as we age, we have to exercise more – a difficult task when so many different things are pulling at our time. If you won't make the time, it just won't happen. We've got to commit to make the time and the right choices, but it seems that all the easy choices are usually the wrong choices. Fast foods are usually high in calories and not nutritious, so you have to prepare a little bit more. I've done all those things personally. Luckily, I have the will power to not pick up bags of cookies, since I have the ability to eat an entire bag if it's in front of me. It isn't hard for me to not buy them, but if they're there, I'll eat them. I can almost hear them calling my name.

Is it just me, or do people ask, Oh my God, I have to do this FOREVER?

It's not just you, but I do think most people who come in are not naïve to dieting. They've usually been on diets on and off for their whole lives, so I try to tell them what they are about to face are *permanent* lifestyle changes. You need to remember that the bypass or the sleeve are permanent fixtures in your life and you're going to use that tool forever to help you keep the weight off. If you don't, and if you revert to your old habits, you're going to put all the weight back on. The act of chewing your food well may slow you down, but it doesn't change the way your brain senses hunger. You may be thin, just like if you've lost a hundred pounds on some severe diet, but your brain doesn't change and doesn't allow you to stay thin. You'll rebound back. You may wish that this were a temporary fix with results that last forever, but in fact, it is not.

I'm a little apprehensive about how my relationship with my spouse might change. What do your patients report?

What many people don't realize is that these weight loss surgeries are major life events, just like marriage, graduation and deaths. They sort of shake things up, including relationships. Most people, as they lose weight, do wind up feeling better about themselves. What often happens for people who are in less than satisfying relationships, however, is that after surgery they may feel that they can do better, and they may find the grass is greener on the other side of the fence. In addition, we see some partners who are threatened because now their husband or wife is more attractive and getting more attention. If you have a strong relationship, then you'll do fine, but if you have a weak relationship, you're more at risk of the surgery causing instability. Plus, one huge source of emotional support is gone. Now that you can't run to food for support, you're going to need a lot more from your partner, and if that's not forthcoming for any reason, that could cause problems.

Do you also hear about a change in their sex lives?

Many people are comfortable dealing with sex at any weight and they're comfortable large or small. Then there are people who are insecure about their weight, so losing weight gives them greater self-esteem. There is also the group of people who, when they were significantly overweight, tell us that they were invisible, and once they lost weight, they suddenly got more attention, and many may exploit their newfound popularity. The bottom line is that people tend to have more or better sex when they're more self-confident and happy, and losing the kind of weight our patients do accomplishes that, plus they report they're getting more offers!

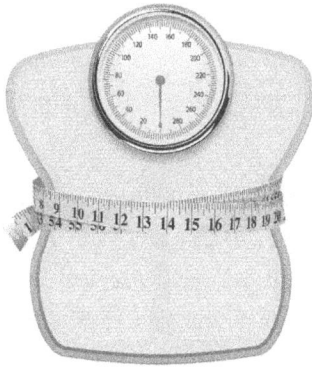

A Bit about Bypass,
a Sliver about Sleeves...

*While gastric bypass has long been considered the gold
standard of weight loss surgeries, we're also getting very good
results with the sleeve gastrectomy. They're both big pieces of
surgery, but they give you the best overall chance of putting the
brakes on the ravages of unchecked obesity. These are by no
means all the questions you'll have about these procedures, but
like the rest of the questions in this book, we hope you will use
them as a little push, a jumping off point for conversations with
your own physician...in other words, your own Weighty Issues.*

Do the bigger patients tend to go for bypass?

We try to recommend it for them and here's why: We standardize height and weight through the Body Mass Index or BMI, and most band patients will lose about eleven BMI points. That means that if you're very, very heavy, you'll still be very heavy even with the band, so we would likely take that procedure off the menu. Now, of course there are exceptions -- people who have lost all their excess weight -- and they sort of break the norm, but with a bypass, you just about double that weight loss on average, especially in the larger, heavier population. While there are certainly hundred-pound losses with bands, I'm talking about people who have to lose 200 pounds or more. Say a man comes in and he's 5 foot 10 and 400 pounds. If he only loses a hundred pounds with the band, he's still 300 pounds, so even though he's a lot better, he can decrease his risk of illness much more if he loses more weight. And for most people, that's with the bypass, especially if, for any reason, they are not candidates for the sleeve gastrectomy.

The sleeve actually began as a staging operation for the bypass, that is, allowing people to get some initial weight off before completing the second stage of the procedure. Many patients, however, had such good results with the sleeve, they didn't need or want anything further. And today, most people opt for that procedure as a stand-alone operation.

So, up to that 50 BMI point, the surgeries are pretty much interchangeable. However, people who achieve those larger sizes – super morbidly-obese with BMIs over 50 – have brains and bodies that are more adept at collecting calories. They find ways to get 'em and keep 'em, and we find bypass usually works best for them in the long run. Plus, bypass offers the best relief for those who suffer from reflux, since food dumps right into the small intestine.

I've met people who are coming back for another type of surgery. Why is that?

Some patients are not satisfied with the weight loss they've achieved with the first operation or they have developed complications – like reflux – that are hampering their lives. We do, however, try to focus on surgical choices early and make careful recommendations as to what might be the best procedures for individuals.

For some people it comes down to risk. The operations where you cut things and reroute things are just inherently a little bit riskier by their nature than ones where you don't, so many of these patients don't want to take that step. They're willing to stick their toe in the pool but they're not ready to just jump in completely. They may pick something simpler and easier like the band, even though we may say *you know, based on what you're telling me about yourself, bypass would be better. It's going to give you more help.* They'll say *no, I can't do that, I can't assume that risk. I have kids, I can't take that much time off work, I'm just not willing to do that.* So if they don't do well with the band, just as we had anticipated, a couple of years later a lot of those people show up wanting to go for the sleeve or all the way to bypass and say *OK, now I'm ready to fix these health problems that didn't go away.* We try to convince people not to go through that succession and choose the best option at the beginning, but it's a personal choice, so we're not going to force that on them. It really depends on how willing you are to work with the system, and then there's some variation with how your body cooperates. Certain drugs have an effect too, which is why for someone who is a severe diabetic, we might say bypass is a little bit better. Some of the drugs you take to treat diabetes make you put on weight, and anyone who's taken them knows this. Most people on oral medication tend to put on weight, especially if they're on insulin. It's sort of a Catch 22. If you lose weight, you improve your diabetic numbers, but the medication works counter to that.

Do bypass and sleeve patients have to eat little bites and chew like crazy forever or does that ease up over time?

They still have to really chew their food, but the restriction is a little bit less than it was with a band, so while they may find they can carefully eat things like bread, sandwiches will be an unlikely choice. You want that pouch to stay small and you want that opening between the stomach and the small intestine in the bypass to stay small, so you're always going to have some difficulty. It becomes second-nature after a short time, so you'll hardly notice it at all.

I've heard many bypass and sleeve patients refer to the honeymoon period, almost longingly. What is it?

The honeymoon period is that first blush of excitement when it seems effortless to lose weight. A lot of people experience a honeymoon period with any new diet regime. They're excited to start it, they're excited to participate, they'll see results quickly and so they're motivated. And then things slow down a little bit, so the honeymoon's over and they want to give up. With both the sleeve and bypass operations, the honeymoon period is really the first six months when you have absolutely no hunger, it's hard to eat a lot of food, you have really little interest in food and you lose weight very rapidly. There are positive things about that and there are negative things, but it seems really easy. After a year-and-a-half or two, you can start eating some of those liquid calories again, ice cream doesn't cause the same adverse reaction anymore, your motivation wanes, and you don't see that fifty pounds just drop off like they did a year ago. Even though you may have lost more, the novelty has sort of worn off, you forget what it was like before and you realize *wow, the honeymoon really is over*. You find it's harder to stay on track, harder to ignore the food that was once your friend. That's one of the reasons post-surgery groups are so important. Patients who can relate to each other offer support and keep each other motivated. It really becomes like family.

OK, what exactly is dumping and what causes it?

It's that famous word again that affects so many people who are trying to lose weight – hormones. When you consume simple carbohydrates or fats, or combinations of the two, the very nature of the bypass operation causes these substances to reach the small intestine a lot sooner than they normally would. Liquids dump immediately into the small intestine, and you get a cascade of hormonal reactions that affect how you feel. One of these reactions creates a profound physical response, similar to a panic attack combined with low blood sugar, leaving you generally feeling like crap. Sleeve patients experience this too, though often to a lesser degree.

The symptoms of dumping are pretty unpleasant. You feel shaky, you have a fast heart rate, you start to feel anxious and headachy, you usually break out into a cold sweat, you then can have cramps, the feeling of things rushing through your intestines, then you'll get diarrhea. There is also something called *late dumping*, which is how you feel a little bit later. It's just fatigue and exhaustion, you sort of want to curl up in bed and stay there, and that's the low blood sugar portion of it.

Things that cause it are high sugar and high fat foods, either/or or both, everything you find in junk foods, meaning cookies, cakes, candies, ice cream. So when a chocolate chip cookie gives you this reaction, you'll think twice the next time you're tempted to eat one.

What could go wrong after a bypass or sleeve that would send you to the ER?

Usually after these operations, you're feeling a little bit better every day, so severe pain could indicate that the surgical connections may be breaking down and leaking. When you get leaking of those digestive contents into that sterile space, you get infections starting. And the body's responses to infections are usually a fast heart rate, sweating, fever, pain, not being able to get a deep breath. These things are usually accentuated compared to days before or immediately after surgery, so that would be a reason to come in. Any sudden-onset shortness of breath or increased pain levels are signs that at least your doctor should get a call. After recovery, the most serious thing that would bring a bypass patient to the ER would be twisting of the intestines, causing a bowel obstruction, or bleeding from an ulcer. Of course, if you don't chew your food well and swallow something too big, you may get food stuck in your new plumbing and have some temporary pain or discomfort. You may even need a procedure to fish it out!

Does the body react differently to alcohol after a bypass or sleeve?

Yes, in general, while the stomach absorbs some of the alcohol, the small intestine absorbs it much faster, so when you do a bypass and alcohol can be much more rapidly absorbed in the small intestine, a lot of people can become cheap drunks. Alcohol not only gets into the bloodstream much faster, the concentrations can be much higher, and since it's the concentration of blood alcohol that gives you the effects of intoxication, you can get much drunker much faster after a bypass or sleeve. So we want people to be careful! Of course, alcohol contains a lot of empty calories, so it doesn't hurt to avoid it altogether for a while.

We've all seen well-known people have weight loss surgery and regain the weight...and they have cooks and trainers. What chance do I have at success?

Everyone is an individual and so are the levels of success and commitment we see with any weight loss surgery. With or without outside support like trainers and cooks, I think you have to be committed to yourself. There are always going to be those people who fail, and it's usually because they sabotage themselves one way or another and just stop trying. It's important to remember that all of these operations are vulnerable to liquid calories. If you actively seek detours around whichever operation we use to make you slow down, then you're going to put on weight. And you can definitely drink all your calories, whether it's from alcohol or high-calorie coffee drinks or just orange juice.

*There's a lot of talk about revisions –
the need for subsequent surgeries.
Why do people have a second surgery,
and which way do they usually go?*

There is always the possibility of revision in bariatric
surgery. Bypasses can break, sleeves can break, bands can
break. There are those who will be unhappy with their weight
loss, and will choose to convert to what's considered a more
extreme operation. After a failed band, most patients choose
the bypass or sleeve gastrectomy. Some people are actually
adding a band on top of a bypass, since we very seldom undo
a bypass. Others are looking to add some of the weight loss
drugs that are largely ineffective when used alone to increase
their weight loss. The problem is that most of the drugs don't
lend themselves to long-term use, so while they can jumpstart
you and re-motivate you, they can't be taken forever. So the
short answer to your question (yes, I know it's too late) is that
bands are only revised to bands if the patient has achieved
good weight loss initially and then for some reason, like the
band slips or the pouch dilates, it failed. Otherwise, bypass or
the sleeve are the most common options.

Can you reverse these operations or are patients stuck with their decisions forever?

We can actually reverse a bypass, but in general, we won't. The biggest reason we would have one reversed is if the patient had symptoms of dumping that just wouldn't go away. There are some medications that might help, but let's say that every time you tried to eat anything that had any sort of fat or any sugar in it, you experienced severe symptoms of dumping, you'd say it's not worth it. If you're passing out, if you wouldn't be able to hold a job, if driving has become dangerous, those would be reasons to consider reversing the bypass. If someone had ulcers that would never heal, then sometimes reestablishing the anatomy might be an option. Really severe complications from the operation, not just weight gain, might convince us, but if a patient says *I just don't want to eat this way, I don't want to have to remember to chew my food,* we won't reverse for that. Of course, sleeve gastrectomy patients have a large portion of their stomachs removed, so we can't reverse a sleeve.

How is a stretched pouch diagnosed?

Well, if the pouch is big, patients report that they're hungry, that they can eat more, and sometimes they have reflux. An x-ray study will confirm that the pouch is enlarged or, for a sleeve patient, that the remaining portion of the stomach has stretched. And that's not going to happen until at least a couple of years after surgery. When it would ordinarily take people fifteen minutes to eat a small plate of food, all of a sudden they can eat the same portion size in five minutes. Tests will show that the pouch is bigger, and for bypass patients, the doorway out of the pouch may also be bigger. Hopefully, we'll be able to see the reason behind it. If there is no reason behind it, it usually means that they are adapting with liquids and there's not much we can do surgically to correct it. I know I've mentioned it many times, but if you're drinking your calories, you can usually get around most of the operations.

A lot of people go for what tastes good and so high-fat choices, like cheese or ice cream, are the likely candidates. It's hard to figure out why people go through surgery and all it entails and then behave that way. It comes down to the fact that, even though surgery is a big deal, some people are just accustomed to thinking second-to-second or minute-to-minute rather than day-to-day, week-to-week or year-to-year. They don't see that the benefits are so much greater than that minute when you're starving and just want something that tastes good. Half an hour later they may feel guilty, but they can't let that cascade into *I'm failing, I'm giving up*...that's when they wake up six months later and find they've put all the weight back on and they finally catch themselves.

I keep hearing that you can get osteoporosis from the bypass. Is that true?

You definitely can, and that's one of the criticisms of the procedures. With these operations, you don't absorb calcium as well as you should, and since primarily women are at risk of osteoporosis as they age, these operations make it riskier still, though less so with the sleeve than the bypass. Someone who gets a bypass at age twenty and doesn't take her vitamins or can't stand the taste of the calcium chews could run into problems with osteoporosis at seventy. It is a real issue. Now most of the people might be seventy or eighty years old when osteoporosis hits, but if you're looking at the life expectancy of the morbidly obese, you'll find very few eighty-year-olds who were morbidly obese their entire lives. So you're trading the possibility of some of these late medical illnesses for better health as you get older.

To say it another way, we can say *sure, you may get osteoporosis when you're eighty, but you may not live to be eighty if you stay morbidly obese.* However, we find it more effective to encourage patients to protect themselves by being vigilant with their vitamins and calcium over the years and to have bone studies as they age. And if what they're taking isn't adequate, there are medications available now that can help mineralize bones. It's *not* a case of being malnourished.

Obesity is being malnourished, meaning taking in too many calories. If you get calories without the proper nutrients, that's malnourishment. So it's not just calories you have to watch, it's the calories plus the proper vitamins and levels of nutrients, meaning carbohydrates, proteins, and fats, that will keep you healthy.

What about iron deficiency with bypass and needing to have infusions?

Very few people actually need to have infusions of iron, but sleeve and bypass patients definitely have to supplement their iron because of the difficulty the body has absorbing it after surgery. Women who have heavy periods are especially at risk. You should be aware that you can cause harm to yourself after surgery if you choose to ignore the changes you have to make. Getting lax with vitamins, calcium and iron are high on the list. While the overall risk of all these operations is low, you just have to be a sensible person and remember that *I need to maintain my body a little differently than I did before my surgery.*

How long should I wait before having a baby after a bypass or sleeve?

We advise our patients that they should not plan on getting pregnant for the first two years following surgery. We don't want to take the chance of any babies being born with birth defects because the moms couldn't keep up with the nutritional regimen, leaving their bodies to decide who is the most important – mother or baby.

Will plastic surgery be necessary after weight loss surgery?

If you start out with a lot of extra skin and the elasticity is gone, as the weight is removed from those areas, the skin doesn't necessarily retract, so you may just develop that *Shar-Pei* look. You can wear firming garments to look great in clothes, but many people are still embarrassed out of clothes, so there are operations done by the plastic surgeons to remove all that extra skin. There are head-to-toe types of procedures and then there are targeted ones for the different problem spots. For some people, excess skin results in chronic irritation or rashes that would be best treated by surgical removal. However, while the majority of people do not need nor do they access plastic surgery, it is there if they feel they want it.

Are the sleeve results about the same as a bypass?

In a sleeve gastrectomy, the resulting stomach pouch is very narrow, so the results are generally pretty similar to a bypass. We are, however, still waiting on long-term data since the sleeve is the newest of the most popular procedures. It's popularity quickly surpassed the band, I think, because many patients prefer an operation where there aren't adjustments required, or they're afraid of devices, or if they live in a location where they don't have easy access to their surgeon, it helps that there's not a lot of maintenance required for a sleeve.

Also, the hormone that stimulates hunger, called *ghrelin*, is produced in the part of the stomach we remove, and many patients report a great reduction in appetite, adding to the success of the surgery. If you take handfuls of pills every day, you may actually be able to swallow them whole, whereas with other procedures, you may to have to crush them for the rest of your life. All of those things should be taken into consideration when selecting an appropriate surgery for you.

What about the after effects of the sleeve gastrectomy? Do sleeve patients get dumping like bypass patients?

They may, but not always. It's not going to be as frequent as with bypass, but you still have to be ready for potential dumping with the sleeve because you can still get rapid emptying of liquids into the small intestine, which is one of the mechanisms for dumping.

With the long staple line of the sleeve, isn't there a risk of leakage and infection?

Yes, the leakage rate is at least as great as with a bypass, probably even greater as we start to try to optimize it, that is, fine-tune it for the greatest weight loss. If we leave it pretty big, it's very safe, but then you don't lose as much weight. If we make it very small, the leak rate goes up significantly, and when you leak, you get infections, and your likelihood of being harmed is much greater.

What do you do when the sleeve leaks?

Well, you don't eat for a long time, that's for starters. You're going to be in the hospital for a long time, you may be in the intensive care unit for a long time, and ultimately, you may even have to convert the sleeve to a bypass to salvage it. But for the most part, if it leaks, you're going to have a longer recovery, and it may be life-threatening. Bands are virtually without that risk, and while any surgery has a risk, you are very seldom going to risk your life getting a band for weight loss. There always will be a small but significant risk with a bypass or sleeve. It's major surgery, and so it's surgery to be taken under very strong consideration.

I keep hearing about 'single incision sleeve surgery.' What should I know about it?

Yes, I get a lot of questions about *single incision*, or *robotic sleeve*. The first thing people need to know is that there's nothing special about these operations themselves; it's an attempt to reduce the number of small incisions from several to one or two. The operation itself on the inside *should* be the same and it's important to ensure that the surgeon can still do the same operation on the inside.

In the single incision process, everything is done through one big incision hidden in the crease of the belly button so that nothing shows. However, if the operation where you cut things and rearrange things is compromised because you're limiting yourself to just one incision, you could run into problems. It really depends on the individual's size, stature and particular medical problems. For example, it may be difficult to fix a hiatal hernia with equipment used in single incision. There are limitations on the strength of the equipment, the angles you can create with the staples, whether or not you can sew, and sometimes you don't know what you're facing until you actually get in there.

Cosmetically, one incision sounds better, but since you're doing this for weight loss, if there's any compromise in the operation – meaning the pouch isn't perfect because of the single incision devices or if a hernia goes unrepaired – you aren't doing yourself any favors by using single incision as the main criterion for choosing a location or surgeon.

There is, however, the overall issue of privacy. There still exists a bit of a stigma about this surgery, and if you can hide the incisions in and around the belly button, nobody will know what the patients had done. Because a lot of people still feel guilt or failure if they have to resort to surgery, if we can come up with a way to *safely* do the procedures, then an added benefit will be that people won't need to advertise they've had surgery for weight loss.

*When weight loss stops
long before your goal is reached,
is there any hope of getting
the rest of the weight off?
Will the level of difficulty
resemble what it was
before surgery?*

While maintaining the weight generally isn't hard, getting to an extreme weight loss is going to be difficult, but doable. With bypass and the sleeve, 60% - 70% excess weight loss is an average goal that people achieve initially, so anything more will be much more difficult unless you resort to extreme measures. You're going to be strictly watching what you eat, and even though you may not want to hear this, you're going to have to move more. A lot of people operate on autopilot, generating a menu of liquids and other things that break down easily because it's more comfortable. A lot of times those things have more calories, so just a few hundred extra calories a day are creeping in, and that's what is maintaining the weight or preventing you from losing more. It's frustrating to people who appear to be doing everything right but still aren't losing weight. However, if you were to follow them around 24/7 and measure the foods they were taking in, they're getting more calories than they're reporting or even realize. So as much as a pain as it is, tracking what you're eating is essential to long-term weight loss. Choosing a plan that essentially teaches you what to eat and how much is key to getting you there.

Even if it's difficult, if you're squeezing off half a pound a week, that's twenty-five pounds in a year. You have to look at the downward trend. If you're putting weight on, even though you think you're being very good, that's more frustrating than continuing on that downward trend, no matter how slowly. The biggest mistake that people make in addition to not curtailing the food intake, is failing to exercise. They really don't want to make exercise a permanent component of their new lifestyle, or if they do exercise, they want to do it two days a week, if that. They really don't want to hear that they should be doing it five to seven days a week, representing a burn of a few hundred calories a day, and that adds up to a lot of pounds in a year. The food intake doesn't parallel the exercise.

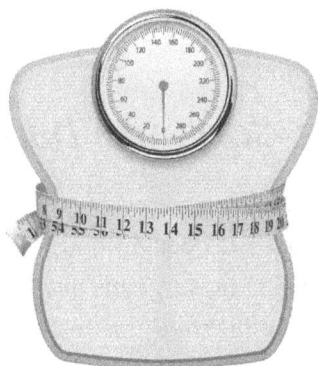

From Bands to Balloons...
and Beyond

When this book was originally published several years ago, lap bands comprised the largest percentage of bariatric surgery procedures for a variety of reasons. They were considered to be minimally invasive, being done laparoscopically, and provided patients with the ability to shed about fifty per cent of their excess body weight. When given the choice of gastric bypass or lap band, many chose the latter. Today, however, lap band has taken a distant third place behind bypass and the sleeve gastrectomy, both of which give patients greater and more enduring weight loss as well as fewer long term complications. So while we've removed a chunk of information about the band and how it works, we realize that hundreds of thousands of patients still have the band, with varying degrees of long term success. That's why we've decided to leave in some of the basic facts about the band while giving you some updated information on what's happening now and what may be in the foreseeable future for weight loss surgery patients.

How long does the band stay in?

Worldwide, banding has been around for about forty years.
When they first put bands in, surgeons put them in with big
incisions. Then, in about the mid-nineties, they started putting
them in laparoscopically, but mostly in Europe, Australia, and
Scandinavia. The band was first approved in the U.S. in 2001
after a thirty-six-month FDA trial. The first FDA-approved
band was the LapBand®, the second was the Realize Band.

That's a long way of saying that the band can stay in
forever. At least that's the intent. Unless there is a pill or a shot
or a new device that is more convenient and allows you to not
have as many interferences in your life like chewing your food
well and eating very small portions very slowly, then it's going
to stay in forever. It has, and it can.

Manufacturers have said, based on their best guess, the
band has a fifteen-year average life span. They've lasted in a
number of people longer than that, but they haven't been in a
lot of people all that long yet. So we don't know if they're
going to last twenty-five years or need to be replaced, or if
there will be a better alternative. The consensus is that fifteen
years from now we'll have something more sophisticated or
simplistic that could take the place of the band...maybe even a
drug.

How will I know when I need an adjustment, or do I just come in every 3000 miles?

Most people need four to five adjustments in the first year, fewer thereafter. Here's why: Imagine a belt. If you're losing weight around your waist, you have to cinch up your belt a notch in order to keep your pants up, but after you've lost a good deal of weight, there won't be a lot of change around the middle. The same thing happens at the top of the stomach. A little bit of the fat melts away, and you have to replace that volume of the fat that's melted away by filling up the band a little. After the first year, the top of the stomach doesn't change as much, so you don't have to continually keep tightening it. You find a spot that's good for you and you work with it there. If you continue to make it tighter, it can be too tight and cause you trouble. Since there are not as many changes going on, there are not as many adjustments needed. You do want to keep your eating at a slow pace so that your brain will get that message to stop, but if you take the detour around the band by eating soup all the time, then you're just making me tighten it more to give you the same effect. The trap people get into is thinking that they'll lose more weight all the time if they're adjusted, meaning having the band made tighter. However, if you can't eat solid food, then you may tend to go to all liquid food. If you choose liquid food that tastes good – and most of the liquid food that tastes good is high-fat and high-calorie – you may even gain weight.

What we really want people to feel a band adjustment does is help them improve satiety, or the feeling of fullness, giving them the power to stop eating within a shorter period of time than they normally would. If they were eating until they were just stuffed, we want them to have the control to stop. We want their hunger to stop, we don't want them to have a band that's so tight that it hurts every time they swallow something, or expect that every time they eat, they'll throw up. So once the steps of eating – chewing your food and slowing down – become habit, eating shouldn't be difficult. You'll just need to follow the rules in order to comfortably stop sooner. By the way, you won't feel the adjustments, you won't actually feel the band tightening or squeezing. What you will feel is a pin prick, much like getting a blood draw, when we access the port under the skin.

When the adjustments stop, plan to see your doctor at least yearly. If you live far away from your surgeon, there can be some partnering with your internist, but you want to make sure he or she has at least the basic knowledge of how the band works and what to look for, and remembers to check your vitamin levels. You need to be doing maintenance on your band for life, because it stays with you for life and you have to be your own advocate. It's much like your car. If the check engine light goes on, you need to check it out. If you hear a funny noise, you don't just turn up the radio and hope it's going to fix itself.

What happens if a band is adjusted too tightly?

Well, if it's really too tight, it'll feel like you're in the middle of a Mortal Kombat game, where someone goes in and grabs the center of your guts and squeezes. If something gets stuck, you'll come to recognize what that feels like. But if a band is too tight, nothing is going to go through, liquids aren't going to go through, you'll have pressure in the center of your chest, you'll have pain and you'll be vomiting. If it's really overfilled, if you've got the maximum volume in there, it's going to feel like someone is squeezing your insides tightly and there will be a lot of pain. But for the most part, if a band's too tight, you just experience an inability to eat certain foods and you're throwing up more often. That's when we may just have to take some of the fluid out. Please note that it does become an emergency if you can't swallow water or your own spit. Get your doctor on the phone or get yourself to the ER.

Does an "overadjusted" band ease up over time?

It can if you lose weight. While it may seem counter-intuitive, if all you can do is drink liquids – and you choose high calorie liquids – you can actually put on weight. But you have to remember that in general, if you lose weight, you lose it all over your body. The top of the stomach generally has some fat tissue on it so as it melts away, the opening increases in size and you can eat a little more. That's when a lot of people whose bands were too tight a month or two ago now may say *I can eat more, I'm hungrier sooner* and require an adjustment. If the top of the stomach shrinks to the extent that the band is now loose, you may benefit from an increased tightening in the future. However, when I told that to one patient whose band may have been slightly overfilled, her reply was *ok, you can go ahead and schedule me sometime between when donkeys fly and when hell freezes over!*

What happens if you get food caught in the band?

You throw up.

I heard about a patient who regained all her weight and went back for gastric bypass, but all she does every day is drink soda.

First of all, no bubbles. That's one of the first rules you learn. Secondly, all liquids should have little or no calories. The only thing about gastric bypass that may help her with long-term behavioral changes is the prospect of dumping. With bypass, if she tries to drink soda with sugar, she'll get really sick, so she'll have a couple of years to learn that *Pepsi is not good in my life, it shouldn't be in my life, it doesn't have to be in my life.* But if she doesn't take that seriously, she'll find that she's now had two major operations that only gave her a relatively short period of time of being thin. It's not worth the risk of surgery if you're not going to have some long-term weight loss, which you need to sustain in order to get the health benefits. Controlling hypertension and diabetes requires long-term lack of excess weight, not just overnight. That's where you have to have commitment. If she continues the behavior after gastric bypass, someone may have to tell her sorry, there are no other options for her. If she were my patient, I just might be that guy.

What kinds of food will I no longer be able to eat?

You will be able to eat almost anything IF you cut your food into very little pieces, chew the heck out of it and eat very slowly. *Almost* is the operative word here. Bread is generally too soft and tends to get stuck in the band, so sandwiches are probably a thing of the past. Sticky rice is problematic, so sushi will no doubt give way to sashimi, which is not such a bad trade. Salads are a little tricky unless they're well-chopped. Red meat doesn't go down as easily as chicken or fish. Other than that, it's pretty much trial and error. If there's something you can't tolerate, believe me, you'll find out in pretty short order.

With some sources saying that the band is not as effective as the bypass or sleeve, do you think the band is everything it was cracked up to be?

I guess the best way to answer that question is this: We know the optimal treatment for weight loss is a moving target. We're committed to bringing the newest, the best, the most improved methods to achieve weight loss. The band is still a safe, effective way of losing weight and maintaining the loss. We know it doesn't consistently achieve the greatest weight loss. We will try to individualize what people are going to use as strategies to achieve weight loss for all the available surgeries. As surgeons, we assess the pluses and minuses of each of these procedures to try to help patients choose the right one. While we know that an average gastric bypass or sleeve patient will probably lose more weight than one with a band, we routinely find individuals with a band who have outdone the other group on average. The reason for trying some of these newer procedures is that no procedure is perfect. We, as the American society, love the newest and the best, and each of these procedures has its own specific strengths and weaknesses. Safety is a major factor and the band is still a very safe way to get the weight off for patients who qualify.

Most people don't need to lose every single pound of excess weight in order to get their health back, and so you can do what you need to do very safely with the band – maybe 40% excess weight loss. If a bypass gives you 70%, it may not make you any healthier than the band does, it may only give you the external appearance of having lost more weight. And while there's certainly something to be said for that, if you're the unlucky person who just so happens to have had a complication when you try to achieve greater weight loss, then you've experienced greater risk than necessary to achieve your benefit.

The data constantly changes as procedures emerge that are safer, more durable and more effective, so at this stage of the game, the consensus is to move toward the newer procedures.

What about the newer gastric balloons? How do they differ from the other surgical procedures?

The balloon is a device that is used to fill a portion of the stomach. There are several different types but they're all volume devices, that is, they all take up certain volume in the stomach by filling it. Some of the balloons are filled with water, others are filled with gas. There are arguments about the pluses and minuses of what the balloons are filled with, but the idea is that by taking up a lot of the volume in the stomach with the device, you can eat less to feel full. People have the most experience with the water-filled balloons. There are several balloon devices out there, but in broadest categories, there are some that have one balloon, others have two – or even three. That's because it is thought that with multiple balloons, it is possible to approximate the shape of the stomach better than with just one. The stomach is not a circle like a balloon, it has more variability in its shape so having two or three balloons might allow it to fit better, be more comfortable. Also, if a balloon pops, you don't want it to go downstream and clog up the plumbing, so having two connected is thought to be the safer design. Balloons are meant to be a temporary implant, lasting about six months, and then they have to come out. Ideally, they should be coupled with what every good weight loss plan should have, which is eating healthy, adding exercise, basically having a healthy lifestyle associated with the device to aid in weight loss. So you're supposed to be doing your part to learn to eat well and lose weight with the help of the device, and when the balloon comes out, continue with these behaviors for the rest of your life.

When the initial studies were done to determine the success of this method, patients were only monitored for one year, but they should anticipate following these behaviors for the rest of their lives if they don't want to gain the weight back.

Do balloon patients really learn how to exercise portion control?

They do. This device is really for a different class of patients than most of the other weight loss surgeries. There are people who are 20 or 40 or 50 pounds overweight and then there are people who are 200 or more pounds overweight, and of course, everything in between. While we couldn't consider a balloon for someone who is 200 pounds overweight, if a patient had 40 pounds to lose, for example – that's sort of the sweet spot for balloon patients – their physiology isn't as messed up or perturbed as the people who need to lose 200 pounds, so they wouldn't need as much in order to achieve the weight loss that would benefit their health.

However, we've talked before about people who just need to lose 10% of their body weight, so if a person weighed 200 pounds, for example, that's a 20-pound loss, and they will get a lot of benefit from that. They might still be overweight, and while it would be better if they lost 50 pounds or so, that 20 pounds can make a huge difference in their health without the need for the full-blown surgery in order to maintain a benefit.

Don't you believe that those who CAN eat more generally do?

If the body's basic physiology hasn't changed, and it's the same as it was a year ago, you'll have a set point that the body anticipates and it's eventually going to float back up to that set point. You can change it a little bit by managing your environment as well as the types of foods you're choosing, but the body is pretty much on auto-pilot, so with the balloon, it's more likely if you don't do something to supplement it, you're probably going to gain the weight back over time. This is a less invasive procedure, you're not making major changes to your body, you're not cutting things, you're not removing things, you're not rearranging things. The balloon may wind up to be something that you can do multiple times. Let's say you do the balloon, it comes out in six months, and a year later, you start to gain some weight. You can put a balloon back in. There's really nothing wrong with that strategy other than it's going to cost you a lot of money because two or three balloons can equal as much as one major surgery, and that major surgery will no doubt carry you through the rest of your life. So the balloon becomes a very costly way to maintain your weight over time.

A lot of people, about 99% of those who qualify for surgery, are not accessing care. They may think for some reason that whatever we're offering is just too much for them. So the balloon is much more attractive to that 99% of the population who aren't accessing any surgical help at all right now.

I'm talking about people who have a body mass index that falls somewhere between 30 and 40. The balloon is less invasive, it's not permanent, it probably isn't going to lead to permanent, long-term weight loss, but many people have lost considerable weight in six months and kept much of it off in that first year. However, since obesity is now categorized as a disease with symptoms that could last for the rest of your life, the balloon probably isn't enough, especially if you have an extreme amount of weight to lose.

From Bands to Balloons...and Beyond 147

What are some of the other newer procedures?

One of them, called the AspireAssist, consists of putting a valve and a tube inside your stomach that you can access through the abdominal wall. It allows you to remove from your stomach a certain portion of the meal that you've eaten. This is also coupled with the necessity of chewing your food well and trying to eat healthy most of the time. If you don't chew well, the particles of food will likely be too big to come out through the tube. It works well, the weight loss is pretty good and can rival some of the surgeries, but it has a grossness factor that puts people off when they first hear about it.

Many critics feel that it's just a form of legalized bulimia. You're going to have to flush your stomach and let this mixture go into the toilet. Because it creates a hole from your stomach to the outside world, you can have irritation of the skin caused by the acid made by the stomach that escapes onto the skin. You're always going to have a little button that you can see through a T-shirt or blouse and, of course, it's visible when your clothes are off. Some people decorate them to try to make them more attractive, but they're still there. Now, like the balloon, this is reversible. You can have it pulled out after it's been in there a while and the hole will just close right up, so it's not necessarily a permanent thing like some of the other surgeries.

While that may make it attractive to some people, if you remove it, you will probably gain back the weight you lost. Though this isn't all that common right now, it is something to be more open-minded about, because having diseases like diabetes, hypertension and all the other conditions that go with being overweight can be very debilitating. If people have opinions that this fits into their lifestyle better than other surgeries, it's still a safe procedure and it may be the style that works for them; and if we can get 2 percent of the people to get help, this might be a way to get these individuals out of the clutches of obesity and improve their overall health. It may not be the best option, but it may be advantageous for individuals who just won't consider the other surgical options.

There are also other types of minimally invasive procedures to choose from. There's still the lap band which works pretty well for a good portion of the people as far as laparoscopic surgeries go, though the sleeve and gastric bypass are still better, and other devices are in the process of being tested. There's something called the Vagal-Blocking device, or V-Bloc, which involves putting a nerve stimulator in your stomach which electrically stimulates nerves and gives you satiety (that lack of hunger in the brain). Now anything that resembles a pacemaker and has a lot of electronics and wiring is always more expensive than a piece of rubber. So unfortunately, not only do patients tend to not lose as much weight with that device as they will with our regular surgeries, the devices themselves are expensive and, therefore, the surgeries will also be more expensive. Also, since they are not covered by insurance, most are performed on a cash basis. As such, they aren't as popular an avenue for most people because of the cost, plus the weight loss isn't as dramatic and more post-op adjustments are needed.

What do you think about lowering the recommended BMI (Body Mass Index) number for weight loss surgery from 35 to 30?

I think that if it's tempered and applied appropriately, many people can benefit from it. It's clear that not everyone, depending on ethnic origin or degree of illness, has to hit 35 in order to see benefits from weight loss. They've done studies around the world that show people with BMIs between 30 and 35 who already have diabetes are clearly going to benefit from weight loss. We've also found that several diabetes meds tend to make people gain weight, so patients are really working against a stacked deck. If you give them a safe, effective way to lose weight that is going to treat their illness, that's great. However, those people who have never tried to diet and just want to do it for cosmetic purposes and just happen to have an appropriate BMI may not be appropriate candidates. So while there may be a greater chance of exploitation, a required BMI of 30 will result in a lot of potential benefit for that select group of people with diabetes with low BMIs.

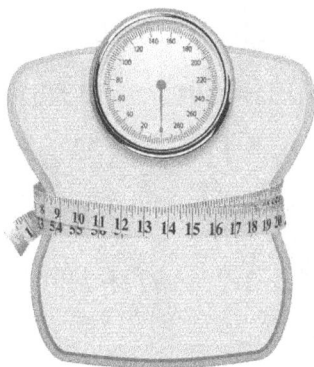

Girl Talk...

*I deal with women in my practice. A LOT of women. I
consider myself pretty tuned-in, but occasionally I hear that
is not necessarily the case. When I was told by one patient,
hey Doc, you WANT to get it, you THINK you get it...but you
just DON'T get it, I called upon Mona Misra, MD, FRCSC,
FACS, FASMBS. She is a bariatric surgeon in private practice
in Beverly Hills, California, and not only does she have a few
more initials after her name than I do, she's a SHE, so we
posed some questions to her. With our profound thanks for her
contribution, here are Dr. Misra's responses.*

OK...I had surgery and my husband's pants fell off! He just THINKS about losing weight and it happens! What's wrong with this picture?

I wish I could say that there is scientific evidence – other than the amount of lean muscle mass in men vs. women – backing up the theory that men tend to lose weight more easily than women, but there isn't. I believe, however, that it has a lot to do with our behaviors. While men often combine volume and speed with comfort-eating, women generally tend to be more sweet-craving, emotional eaters. Most of these sweets are in the liquid calorie category (chocolate, ice cream, etc.), and therefore are not stopped or affected by the restrictions of weight loss surgery.

Most of the women I see admit to emotional eating, but it's also the type of foods they're eating that's a problem – more sweets, more high-calorie comfort foods. With surgery, we can't control WHAT you eat, only that you eat smaller portions. We aim for satiety, feeling full with less food, but we can't stop you from wanting sweets. Snickers are Snickers, before or after surgery. Whatever hormone changes she's going through in whatever stage of life she's in, chocolate is always going to make a woman feel different than it would a man. There is a reason why most chocolate commercials have women looking like they are in heaven as they eat a bite of chocolate. We women can relate to that. Surgery will not necessarily stop that feeling, but giving in to it may cause dumping syndrome in gastric bypass and some sleeve patients. All we can do is try to understand why we are reaching for the chocolate/sweets and try to change those patterns to make a difference. And remember, I'm not saying you can't ever have chocolate... you can, just SMALL amounts infrequently, not a daily indulgence.

Do hormones inhibit weight loss?

Well, yes and no. Some researchers have found a correlation between estrogen and weight *gain*, particularly during menopause, when estrogen levels drop. While there is no specific evidence to show that hormones (like estrogen) adversely affect weight *loss*, I do believe that hormones can affect emotions. We know that obesity and weight loss are physical and psychological battles, so it seems to make sense that if hormones affect cravings (such as sweets or carbohydrates like potato chips), this will, in turn, affect or inhibit weight loss.

While there may not be real science behind what I'm saying, it's an opinion based on anecdotal evidence, and a pattern I definitely see in my practice.

When women stop losing weight after surgery, are they on their own and back to square one to lose the rest of the weight?

The surgery will give you the tools that will correct your health problems, helping you to lose probably 50%-60% of your excess body weight. If you still want to lose additional weight, whether for health, comfort, or cosmetic purposes, that's when diet and exercise need to kick in to really make a difference. We understand that initially surgery was needed because if you were a hundred pounds overweight and if someone told you to *go on a diet and go for a run,* you probably wouldn't be able to do that. It would be like *me* riding on your back. It would be very hard on your knees, your hips, all your joints, making it very uncomfortable, if not painful. Once some of the weight is lost, though, it is physically easier to exercise and you will have more energy, so you need to take advantage of that and exercise. We understand it's not necessarily that you are consuming more calories than anyone else. What you have to realize is that even if you're taking in only one hundred additional calories each day, that can represent almost a ten-pound gain in a year. You need to make sure that you are burning more calories than you are consuming. That's why diet and exercise will get you to that next level and keep you there. Plus, after having lost the initial weight, the exercise will be easier and more effective, and you'll be able to stick with it. So yes, you're pretty much on your own, but now with the knowledge and the tools to help you succeed like you never did before.

My weight fluctuates constantly. It's SO frustrating. What can I do?

Don't be a slave to the scale. Don't focus on that one to two pounds you'll see because of the time of the month or a birthday dinner. It's clothing size and energy level that matter. *Comorbidity resolution*, that's what you want. The scale will *always* lie. You get constipated, the scale goes up. You ate Chinese food last night, the scale goes up. Those pounds don't matter on a day-to-day basis. Keep your eye on the finish line.

What can women do to preserve whatever elasticity is left in their skin when they lose so much weight?

Exercise makes a big difference. You're always going to have a little bit of give when you lose a lot of weight, but exercise will help you tone it up a little bit. If you prefer to be tight after all your weight is lost, plastic surgery tummy tucks can help with that. We do recommend waiting until all your weight is lost, though, otherwise you will likely need the process more than once…and why waste the money or subject yourself to additional surgery? Significant excessive skin, however, can actually become a medical problem, and that's when we refer patients to plastic surgeons.

Where did those boobs go?

Sorry to tell you this, but your weight is going to be lost *everywhere*. Unfortunately, wherever you have fat, that's where you are going to lose it. It comes off of your face, it comes off of your neck, it comes off of your fingers. If it disappears from that place you don't want it to, just remember...that's why we have places like Victoria's Secret! ☺

Should women be given a different set of instructions after surgery than men?

The instructions may not differ, but the support system definitely should because following surgery is where the emotional component comes in. It must be tailored to the patient's needs. I have found women usually need a little more emotional support than men do because society puts a lot more pressure on women to be losing that weight. With men, it seems to be more acceptable if they're a little larger…for them it's called *husky*…just like men can be a little older and it's no big deal, they look *distinguished*, but women are held to a different standard. We can get so defeated, trying to fit into society's ideal of what women should look like. There is a lot of evidence showing many patients suffering from depression and obesity, so we need to be sensitive to their complex needs. We provide dieticians, social workers, psychologists, and myself to both our men and women patients. I find my women patients need a little more support and I try to provide whatever they need. A lot of people are coming to surgery as their last resort. They think *I've failed before and if I fail this, I'm doomed* and that's when they need to know that they're not doing this alone this time around. We're here to help and this is something that is actually going to work.

Do you have any tips for women that would make success more attainable?

I think the biggest dilemma I see is making sure the changes in your life are sustainable. Most women are very enthusiastic in the beginning, *I'm going to stick to these rules and I'm going to measure all my food in a cup, count every calorie, exercise constantly,* but all of these changes are so difficult to keep doing forever. I don't want to discourage the behavior when they're so gung ho about it, but I do try to warn them early on that they're not going to be able to do that ten years from now, if they don't make it part of normal life. I worry I'm going to see them two years from now and the likelihood is that they're going to be tempted to cheat, so I need them to stick to things they can actually do. It's great if you can work out five days a week, and this is something you can do as long as you incorporate it into your routine life. You're not going to be working out eight hours a day like they used to on shows like *The Biggest Loser* and so when you stop working out, or watching what you are eating, you likely will put some weight back on, and you're going to be disappointed and pissed off and frustrated that you were not able to maintain it. So I try to tell people to do things that are actually going to be easier for them to do.

That's why watching portion sizes helps, keeping in mind a rough idea of calories – so about 300-400 calories for a meal (that's like a piece of chicken, some rice and some vegetables), and 100 calories for a snack (yogurt or a protein bar). You can actually do that as opposed to counting out every single thing you put in your mouth, thinking *oh my God, what am I eating*, because trying to do that forever is going to be really hard. I try to think of myself, and I know people laugh because I'm really tiny, but you know, everybody has to battle this, even people who have that great metabolism. There is a constant keeping track of what you're doing, and I know if I had to count every single thing all the time, it would drive me crazy forever.

I'd feel as if I'm always on a diet and wouldn't really enjoy food, so I really want you to enjoy this process and not keep thinking, *ok, what do I eat now?* That's too stressful. Food is an addiction, so it can always be in the back of your head. It's like, *oh look, it's those little cake pops, I want to try one of those,* and being faced with those temptations and making changes in your life is hard, so start slowly, changing one thing at a time. Start with one walk for fifteen minutes a day, three times a week to begin with, and go from there, increasing frequency and length of time.

I also think that keeping it real is so important. Rather than being a slave to the scale, know for yourself where you want to be, something that's realistic, not just what some insurance company chart says you should be.

What do you want women to know before they leave your office?

First of all, if you go through this process and have this idea that you're going to look like a supermodel or movie star, you have to realize that many of these Hollywood ideals are *plastic surgeried-out*. They've had things added and subtracted and moved around...and that is not your goal. You want to be comfortable in your own body. Nobody fits into one shape. Everyone's shape is different and you have to find what is right for you. You're doing this for yourself, not for someone else, so only you can decide what is the proper weight for you to feel comfortable and healthy. A lot of people think *I've got to find somebody or I've got to keep someone with me,* and that's not what it's about. It's not about comparing yourself with your friends, either. It's all about *you*...and not just about trying to look a certain way. Now, if that's one of your goals, that's great, but your main goal should be to live long and to live well. It's not enough to be eighty years old living your life on an oxygen tank, losing your feet from your diabetes, right? It's about living longer, healthier, and loving yourself!

When my patients tell me *I don't have time to make a snack for myself in the middle of the day because I'm too busy,* I tell them *if you die of a heart attack five years from now, is your boss going to say, oh that girl, she was so great because she never took a five-minute break for a snack?* They don't care if you take a tiny break! You have to do it for yourself! A lot of my patients have raised their kids and lived their lives thinking *everyone else comes first and I come last.* Most of us do take care of everyone else first and ourselves last. But priorities have to change. *You* have to matter, and I think realizing that is a big part of changing your priorities. You're doing this for yourself to live long and live well, and you have to remember that *you're important.* So taking time for yourself is important, and if you say *there's no way I'm going to be able to make this happen,* I'm telling you *yeah, you can!*

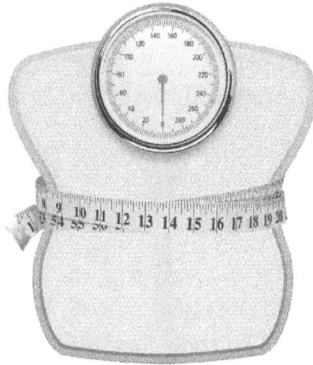

The Last Word...

Dr. Cunneen, if there's one thing you'd like us to take away from these conversations with you, what would it be?

You may have noticed by now that I'm not the kind of guy who can limit my thoughts to *one thing*, but I'll give it a try. Your health is at stake. Being severely overweight threatens your life every day, maybe a little bit at a time, maybe *bam*, the big one. *You've* got to make the decision to determine the quality of your own life. *You've* got to make the commitment to change your attitude, your lifestyle, your relationship with food...forever. If that decision includes weight loss surgery, we hope we have contributed in some small way to the information you need to make these important choices. We wish you good health.

Dr. Scott Cunneen

The Questions...

NOTES

www.ingramcontent.com/pod-product-compliance
Lightning Source LLC
Chambersburg PA
CBHW031200270326
41931CB00006B/351